Lifetime Fitness

Lifetime Sport and Fitness Series

Lifetime Fitness

Second Edition

H. Larry Brown
North Carolina State University

Contributing Authors:

Sally Almekinders

Lynn Berle

Donna Clark

Kathy Davis

Jim DeWitt

Tom Evans

Bob Gwyn

Charles Raynor

Tom Roberts

Timothy Winslow

George Youtt

Gorsuch Scarisbrick, Publishers
Scottsdale, Arizona

Consulting Editor for the Lifetime Sport and Fitness Series: Robert P. Pangrazi,
Chairman of the Department of Physical Education • Arizona State University

Editor: John W. Gorsuch
Consulting Editor: Robert Pangrazi
Production Manager: Carol Hunter
Cover Design: Gordon Fong, The Omni Group
Typesetting: Carlisle Communications, Ltd.

Gorsuch Scarisbrick, Publishers
8233 Via Paseo Del Norte, Suite F-400
Scottsdale, AZ 85258

10 9 8 7 6 5 4 3

ISBN 0-89787-613-X

Printed in the United States of America.

Preface

Good health and fitness are the cornerstones of a productive, healthy, and happy life. *Lifetime Fitness* will help you understand the benefits of physical exercise and proper nutrition; the information, figures, and tables in this book are designed to offer the student a concise overview of the many factors contributing to the development and maintenance of a healthy body. The latest scientific information has been used in the discussions of all topics relating to health and fitness.

Lifetime Fitness will help you evaluate your overall level of fitness, including your cardiorespiratory fitness, which plays an essential role in your overall good health. You can then design a personalized exercise program to achieve the fitness goals you set for yourself. Step-by-step instructions for many exercises are included in the book, accompanied by photographs. In addition, the book identifies problems and injuries that may be encountered during training, and suggests safety considerations to avoid them.

Lifetime Fitness discusses the vital role nutrition plays in overall good health, and provides detailed information about nutrients and their functions. Finally, this book includes a chapter on *stress*—the causes, the symptoms, the results, and what you can do to reduce the stress of everyday life.

The health and fitness program you choose today will have a major impact on your future lifestyle. Using the information in *Lifetime Fitness,* you can design a program that will be both fun and productive.

I wish to thank the following contributing authors for their help in making *Lifetime Fitness* the concise, up-to-date book it is: Sally Almekinders, Lynn Berle, Donna Clark, Kathy Davis, Jim DeWitt, Tom Evans, Bob Gwyn, Charles Raynor, Tom Roberts, Timothy Winslow, and George Youtt.

Contents

1
Introduction

Why lifetime fitness? Because it promotes a happier, more fulfilling, productive life. When a brilliant but obese, stress-laden, heavy-smoking, and physically inactive individual is unable to work or dies from a coronary during middle age, a human resource is lost. While it is difficult to prove that being fit will lengthen your lifespan, it is certain that fitness does improve the quality of life. Evidence indicates overwhelmingly that our learning potential, within our given level of intelligence, increases in accordance with our level of physical fitness. A gradual reduction of functional capacity for thought, work, and recreation will occur if you allow yourself to succumb to the ease and comfort of today's electronic push-button world. However, an active lifestyle will enable you to enjoy the comforts of modern technology without losing functional capacity.

Keeping fit and practicing good health habits are your responsibility. Your future health and well-being depend largely upon the lifestyle you are now developing. This book will help you understand the principles of fitness and apply these concepts to your own plan for lifetime fitness.

Physical Fitness

Physical fitness is often defined as the ability to perform daily physical tasks energetically and still have energy reserves to perform recreational activities and respond to emergencies requiring strength and stamina. Fitness is not merely **being well** or **not being sick.** It is a positive quality of life with quantitative graduations ranging from a vigorous and abundant life at one end of the spectrum to death at the other. All people exhibit a state of physical fitness; this state is minimal in the severely ill and of much greater magnitude in the highly conditioned individual.

Very few individuals extend the effort to reach their maximum potentials, although many are able to improve their fitness levels. A common fallacy is to equate athletic ability, the ability to perform specific sport skills, with physical fitness. It is true that the majority of highly trained athletes are physically fit, but this does not imply you must possess athletic ability to achieve a high level of fitness. Many individuals who have attained high fitness levels through regular participation in well planned fitness programs are not, and never have been, skilled athletes. There are also numerous examples of individuals who have mastered certain athletic skills and yet are not physically fit.

Components of Fitness

The four components of fitness are **flexibility, cardiorespiratory capacity, muscular strength,** and **muscular endurance.**

Flexibility.   Flexibility is the functional capacity of a joint to move through a normal range of motion. Flexibility is highly specific and depends largely upon the muscles and connective tissue *surrounding* the joint. (Though arthritis and other bone diseases certainly affect the joint itself.) Good flexibility is characterized by freedom of movement and contributes to ease and economy of muscular effort.

Cardiorespiratory (CR) Capacity.   Cardiorespiratory (CR) capacity is the functional capacity of the heart, lungs, and blood vessels to take in and deliver oxygen to the aerobic working muscles. Generally, CR fitness is developed through involvement in sustained activities such as running, swimming, cycling, rowing, cross-country skiing, and others that require the use of large muscle groups in rhythmic fashion.

Muscular Strength.   Muscular strength is the maximum amount of force a muscle or group of muscles can exert during one contraction. Muscular strength, in its purest form, is utilized in activities requiring maximum force to be exerted in a single, all-out effort. Lifting a barbell one time with as much weight on it as you can lift is an example. Most activities, however, require more than a single maximum effort and are a combination of muscular strength and endurance. It should be noted that in many fitness programs test items used for measuring muscular strength in fact measure a combination of muscular strength and endurance.

Muscular Endurance.   Muscular endurance is the ability of a muscle or group of muscles to exert force for an extended period of time. Strength and muscular endurance are directly related but are at opposite ends of the strength-endurance training continuum. The more times a muscular movement is repeated the closer it is to the endurance end of the continuum.

A good fitness program includes activities that will develop all fitness components. Adequate rest and a balanced diet must also be included to obtain desired results. Practically anyone can become fit; the only requirements are time and dedication.

Entrance Evaluation

You should evaluate your present condition prior to participating in a regular fitness program. Identify any medical problems you may have; if you have any medical problems or are over the age of 35, you should receive a medical examination before beginning a fitness program. If you have no medical restrictions, evaluate yourself on a few performance tests to establish your fitness level in regards to the four components of fitness.

Flexibility.   Many tests are used to measure flexibility. One of the most important is the **sit and reach test,** which measures the flexibility of the lower back and hip extensors. Lack of flexibility in these areas, combined with poor strength in the abdominals and hip flexors, can lead to chronic back pain. The procedures for administering the test are found in Chapter 3, and the norms are listed in table 3.1.

Cardiorespiratory (CR) Capacity.   The most accurate method to determine the cardiorespiratory fitness of an individual is to measure the oxygen consumption using a graded exercise stress test. However, this method is both time-consuming and costly. Therefore, the **step test** and the 1.5 mile run are often used when testing large groups of young, healthy college students.

The step test consists of stepping up and down on a bench, the height of which is 14 inches for women and 18 inches for men, at a rate of 120 steps per minute for 3 minutes (time 0:00 to 3:00). The movement of each foot, up or down, counts as one step. At the end of three minutes, the participant sits down and locates the radial pulse (on the inside of the wrist) within 10 seconds (time 3:01 to 3:10). It is beneficial to have another counter find the carotid pulse (above the collarbone to either side of the Adam's Apple) while you are finding the radial pulse. It is extremely important that the individual taking the carotid pulse does not press down firmly or the blood supply to the brain may be decreased. The pulse count is then taken for 15 seconds (time 3:11 to 3:25) and recorded. You then prepare to take the pulse again. The pulse is taken twice more (from time 4:11 to 4:25 and from 5:11 to 5:25). Normally, the fitter you are, the lower each score will be. Also, if you exercise regularly, the change between the first and second counts will be greater than the change between the second and third counts. Norms for the step test for college students are given in tables 1.1 and 1.2.

The time period it takes to run 1.5 miles is often used to measure cardiorespiratory fitness. It is advisable to use the step test rather than the 1.5 mile run as an entrance evaluation method if you are not moderately conditioned before entering a fitness program. In many fitness programs, the 1.5 mile run is not utilized as an entrance test because of the difficulty untrained individuals have in judging pace. The norms for the 1.5 mile run are listed in table 4.1 in Chapter 4.

Muscular Strength.   As mentioned earlier, muscular strength is the maximum amount of force that can be exerted during one contraction. A valid test of muscular strength is the bench press. To test yourself, read the instructions in Chapter 5 and look at figures 5.1 and 5.2. Find the weight that you are sure you can press more than one time. Use spotters and press the weight as many times as possible. Do not hold your breath while lifting. After determining how many times you can lift a particular weight, you need to compute the maximum weight you could have lifted one time. To compute the maximum weight, use the Brown formula: Maximum Weight = [(Repetitions $\times$ .0328 + .9849) $\times$ Resistance]. For example, if you lifted a weight of 150 pounds six times, you would compute your maximum weight: [(6 $\times$ .0328 + .9849) $\times$ 150] = 177 pounds. Tables 1.1 and 1.2 list the norms for college age students. To determine how you compare against other college students, compare the maximum weight you can lift to your body weight. For instance, in the example above your maximum weight was 177 pounds. If you weigh 140 pounds, the ratio of your maximum weight compared to your body weight will be 177:140, which gives you a ratio of 1.26. According to table 1.1, this would place you within the 80–90 percentile.

Muscular Endurance.   A test often used to determine muscular endurance is the one minute sit-up. In this test you perform as many bent-knee sit-ups as possible in one minute. The hands should be crossed across the chest, knees bent at a 90 degree angle, and the feet flat on the floor. Start in a supine position on the floor with the knees bent at a 90 degree angle. Perform the sit-up by flexing the trunk to raise the trunk upward to the sitting position with the elbows touching the knees. Return to the starting position. Repeat the exercise as many times as possible during a one minute period. Keep the hips flat against the floor. See figures 5.37 and 5.38. Norms for college age students are listed in tables 1.1 and 1.2.

Height, Weight, and Percent Fat.   In addition to measuring the four components of fitness upon entering a fitness program, it is also recommended that you measure height, weight, and percent body fat. Since your height and weight are measured throughout your life, we will assume that you understand how to measure these items.

The procedure for measuring your percent body fat is given in Chapter 7 and the norms are listed in table 7.1. Tables 7.2 and 7.3 can be used to help you determine your percent fat.

Test Results and Their Meanings

The norms for the preceding tests for college students are listed in tables 1.1 and 1.2. This information will allow you to compare your test results to those of approximately 36,000 young men and 9,000 young women tested at North Carolina State University.

These results will give you a starting point to maintaining a progression record. You should not be concerned about the percentile you are now in. However, it is important to keep track of your performance level as you progress. Be concerned with your goals, and not with your past record.

Supplementary Readings

1. Allsen, P. E., J. M. Harrison, and B. Vance. *Fitness for Life*. Dubuque, IA: Wm. C. Brown, 1989.
2. Harris, Dorothy V., and James A. Peterson. *Personal Fitness Guide*. Englewood, CO: Morton Publishing Company, 1988.
3. Hoeger, W. K. *Lifetime Physical Fitness and Wellness*. Englewood, CO: Morton Publishing Company, 1988.
4. Marley, W. P. *Health & Physical Fitness*. Dubuque, IA: Wm. C. Brown, 1988.
5. Mazzeo, Karen. *A Commitment to Fitness*. Englewood, CO: Morton Publishing Company, 1985.

TABLE 1.1 Entrance evaluation norms—Men.

Percentile	Sit-ups	Bench*	Step EoT	Step + 1	Step + 2
99	60	1.60	15	12	12
90	48	1.32	30	22	19
80	45	1.20	33	24	21
70	43	1.12	34	26	22.5
60	41	1.05	35	27.5	24
50	38	.99	36.5	29	25
40	37	.93	37.5	30	27
30	36	.87	38.5	32	27.5
20	33	.81	40	34	28.5
10	28	.74	41.5	41	30.5

For the bench, the value is the ratio of the maximum weight one can lift to his body weight.

TABLE 1.2 Entrance evaluation norms—Women.

Percentile	Sit-ups	Bench*	Step EoT	Step + 1	Step + 2
99	44	.735	18	13	12.5
90	30	.520	33	22.5	19.5
80	28	.488	35	26	22
70	26	.462	36	27.5	24
60	24	.438	37	29	25.5
50	23	.419	38	30	26.5
40	22	.400	39	31	27.5
30	20	.380	40	32.5	29
20	19	.354	41	33.5	29.5
10	17	.322	42.5	35	31

For the bench, the value is the ratio of the maximum weight one can lift to her body weight.

Note: For tables 1.1 and 1.2
   EoT refers to pulse count at end of test.
   + 1 refers to pulse count one minute after completion of test.
   + 2 refers to pulse count two minutes after completion of test.

2
Safety and Training Considerations

This chapter will identify training principles and guidelines that should be considered before participating in a training program. Careful attention to these principles and guidelines will maximize results from the training program, and maintain safety.

As mentioned in Chapter 1, if you are over the age of 35 years or have any medical problems, you should receive clearance from a physician before participating in an exercise program. It is also important to consider your physical limitations when deciding on the type of activities your program will include. For example, if you are overfat, it would be advantageous for you to start with a walking or swimming program before participating in a jogging program.

Training Principles

Correct principles must be incorporated into a training program in order to achieve desired results. These principles include the overload principle, the law of reversibility, and the law of specificity.

Overload Principle. In order for a muscle cell to increase in size (hypertrophy) and strength, the workload must be increased beyond what the cell normally experiences. Furthermore, once a muscle has adapted to a higher workload, additional increases in the workload are required for further strength gains. The overload principle is the underlying concept of progressive resistance training.

Progression Principle. As physiological adaptations from training take place in the body, you will experience a sensation of reduced effort for a given performance. This is due to the adaptations enhancing your ability to remove metabolic by-products and replace energy. In order to continue to overload your system for steady improvement, you should increase your training intensity. This will be a continual process in your training program.

Law of Reversibility.   Even though you may have a high level of fitness, you must continue a regular program of training in order to avoid deconditioning. A significant reduction of working capacity begins to occur within two weeks after cessation of training. The saying *"use it or lose it"* certainly applies to physical fitness. The effects of training are transient and dependent upon continued training. Cessation of training results in a gradual decline of performance capacity and a decrease in size (atrophy) of the adapted muscle cells.

Law of Specificity.   Training is specific to the cells and to the structural and functional elements within the cells that are overloaded. Transfer of training occurs only to the extent that the same motor units are recruited and used in a similar manner. A motor unit consists of a motor neuron with all the muscle cells it innervates. When attempting to increase your muscular strength and endurance for a given activity, it is best to perform the movement required in the activity against resistance. If the nature of the activity does not permit this, then the major muscle groups involved in the activity should be trained using progressive resistance exercises as similar as possible to the movement of the activity. The development of muscular strength and endurance is dependent upon the type and amount of exercise performed.

Training Guidelines

Regardless of the activities selected for use in your program, each training session should be preceded by a warm-up and followed by a cool-down (also referred to as a warm-down). In addition, guidelines with respect to frequency, intensity, and time (duration) need to be set and followed to ensure that the body receives a safe training stimulus during the workout. These components of the training guidelines are often referred to as **"FIT"** (frequency, intensity, time).

Warm-up.   The warm-up consists of an easy whole body activity prior to beginning the workout session. There are three phases in the warm-up: cardiorespiratory, static stretching, and muscular endurance. The warm-up should begin with easy whole body activity to raise the muscle and blood temperature to produce sweating but not so strenuous as to cause fatigue. Static stretching and light muscular endurance exercises should follow. It is especially important that the muscles that will be utilized during the workout are warmed up. A warm-up prior to activity not only prepares the body for participation but also helps to prevent injury.

Cool-down   A cool-down implies a gradual tapering of activity. A good rule of thumb is to slowly taper the intensity level until your heart rate is is below 100 beats per minute. Cooling down tends to prevent pooling of the blood. Static stretching is also part of the cool-down process; it helps to reduce delayed localized soreness and improves flexibility.

Frequency. It is recommended that the body receives a training stimulus every 36 to 48 hours for optimal results in a training program. In strength training, a training stimulus every other day is preferable. In cardiorespiratory activities, training is generally recommended three to five days a week for weight bearing activities such as jogging and running, and five to seven days a week for non-weight bearing activities such as cycling and swimming. Training more than five days a week in the weight bearing activities will often result in overuse injuries. Nevertheless, it is possible to train seven days a week without overuse injuries if a variety of activities are used for cardiorespiratory training. For example, you could swim and jog on alternating days and probably train seven days a week without injuries from overuse.

Attire. Depending upon the activity, the attire for training normally consists of porous, loose fitting clothing, a good pair of shoes, and an identification bracelet or tag. Also, a medical alert tag should be worn if you have medical problems that may need attending in the event you are unable to communicate. Never use rubberized suits or windbreakers, which do not "breathe." Dress so that you do not overheat in the summertime or become overexposed during the winter. During cold weather, you need to protect the head, ears, face, fingers, toes, and genitals. Listen to weather reports and dress accordingly. Protect yourself against foot and knee problems by wearing proper footwear. Also, be aware that many activities require special equipment, such as goggles for swimming.

Environment. Environmental conditions should be considered when structuring your program. These conditions include weather, terrain, altitude, pollution, type of facility, water temperature, and so on. Each of these factors will affect your performance.

In order to avoid dehydration on hot, humid days, it is advisable to drink plenty of fluids and to avoid long training sessions where water may not be available. During the training session, you should drink fluids approximately every twenty minutes and immediately following the workout. Light colored clothing will reflect some of the heat to keep you cooler. Also, during the summer the time of day you train is important. Training in the early morning offers the advantage of cooler temperatures while the evening hours are normally less humid. However, when training during low light hours, be sure to wear reflective clothing or tape to alert motorists to your presence.

The main problems of training in cold weather are frostbite and hypothermia. Frostbite normally occurs to the fingers, toes, penis, nose, and ears. To avoid frostbite of these areas, the individual should dress warmly. Hypothermia can be avoided by dressing warmly and by avoiding extremely low temperatures. Wearing dark clothing will absorb some of the sun's heat.

Environmental pollution is often a problem when training in urban areas. Exercising in high pollution levels may lead to impaired lung function and decreased work capacity. In addition, the toxicity of environmental pollutants are increased during vigorous exercise due to the greater air exchange in the lungs. If you live in a polluted area, it is best to train in the early morning or late evening when the pollutant levels are generally lower. The highest pollutant levels usually occur between twelve noon and six P.M. In addition, you should avoid jogging on roads with heavy traffic or near industrial factories. Dust may also be a problem; it is best to avoid areas with loose topsoil if the weather conditions have been dry and windy.

As the altitude increases, the partial pressure of oxygen decreases, thereby increasing the stress placed on the cardiorespiratory system during vigorous exercise. The human body normally adapts to this stress within ninety days by increasing the hemoglobin levels, which in turn increases the blood's oxygen carrying capacity.

Exercise Program

Your program should consist of activities that you enjoy, and yet provide your body with an adequate and safe training stimulus for cardiorespiratory fitness, flexibility, and muscular strength and endurance. For example, you may want to weight train on Mondays, Wednesdays, and Fridays and play full court basketball on Tuesdays, Thursdays and Saturdays. These activities, preceded by a warm-up and followed by a cool-down, would give you an adequate and safe training stimulus in each fitness component as long as the training guidelines regarding frequency, intensity, and time are followed. Chapters 3, 4, and 5 have more specific information on training for flexibility, cardiorespiratory fitness, and muscular strength and endurance. Remember, in order to develop and/or maintain fitness, you must participate on a regular basis in a program that will develop all four components of fitness.

Nutrition

The results you obtain from your training program will also depend upon your diet. You should not attempt to participate in a training program without providing the essential nutrients for your body. Proper nutrition contributes to the functioning of all bodily processes.

Unfortunately, there is much false information on the market concerning diet and nutrition. Before depriving your body of nutrients by engaging in a fasting or weight loss program, please take time to read the information in Chapters 6 and 7 of this book.

Rest

In addition to adequate exercise and nutrition, the body must receive adequate rest in order to gain or maintain fitness. The body is able to withstand some abuse in regard to exercise, diet, and rest. However, abuse on a regular basis will lead to bad health. Give your body the rest it needs. On the average, people require between six to nine hours of sleep a night.

Supplementary Readings

1. Allsen, P. E., J. M. Harrison, and B. Vance. *Fitness for Life.* Dubuque, IA: Wm. C. Brown, 1989.

2. Harris, Dorothy V., and James A. Peterson. *Personal Fitness Guide.* Englewood, CO: Morton Publishing Company, 1988.

3. Hoeger, W. K. *Lifetime Physical Fitness and Wellness.* Englewood, CO: Morton Publishing Company, 1988.

4. Marley, W. P. *Health & Physical Fitness.* Dubuque, IA: Wm. C. Brown, 1988.

5. Mazzeo, Karen. *A Commitment to Fitness.* Englewood, CO: Morton Publishing Company, 1985.

3
Flexibility

Flexibility is defined as the range of possible movement about a joint. It is an important component of physical fitness but is frequently overlooked or ignored when fitness programs are being planned. The degree of flexibility is determined by the shape of the bones and cartilage in the joint and by the length of muscles and ligaments crossing the joint. The spectrum of flexibility ranges from the contortionist seen at the circus, who is extremely loose jointed, to arthritic patients whose range of movement is severely restricted. Adequate flexibility permits freedom of movement, contributes to the ease and efficiency of muscular effort, and helps to reduce susceptibility to some types of musculoskeletal problems and injuries.

Terminology

Stretch Reflex.   As a muscle reaches a fully stretched position, pain receptors in the muscle sense pain and trigger an involuntary protective response that causes the muscle to contract. Without such an automatic reaction, serious muscle and/or tendon injury due to overstretching could occur.

Antagonist-Stretch.   Muscles are stretched by the force of the contraction of the opposing muscle. For example: when performing the hamstring stretch (figure 3.18), the quadriceps muscles in the front of the upper leg contract to cause stretching of the hamstring muscles in the back of the upper leg.

Dynamic Stretching.   *Dynamic* stretching is characterized by rapid bouncing or jerking movements. An example of dynamic stretching, using the hamstring stretch, would be a series of up and down bouncing movements of the torso as one stretches to touch the toes with the hands (figure 3.18).

Proprioceptive Neuromuscular Facilitation (PNF).   PNF is a method of stretching often employed by athletic teams and in exercise classes. It normally requires a partner and more time than the other methods of stretching. PNF involves a series of contractions and relaxations of the muscle fibers in the muscle group being stretched. Initially, your partner will move your limb which is being stretched partially through its range of movement (figure 3.1). At the angle at which movement is stopped, you should contract isometrically for a period of four to five seconds against the leverage being applied by your partner. Upon completion of the isometric contraction, completely relax and allow your partner to move the limb to a greater angle without discomfort being felt (figure 3.2). The sequence is terminated before discomfort is felt. **Always terminate a stretching exercise before discomfort is felt.**

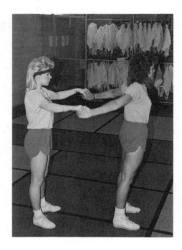

FIGURE 3.1

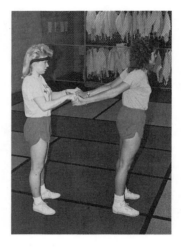

FIGURE 3.2

Static Stretching.   Static stretching, sometimes referred to as passive stretching, is accomplished by slowly stretching a muscle and holding it at greater than resting length for a short period of time. Using the hamstring stretch as an example, static stretching would entail bending at the waist and easing your hands along the front of your legs slowly and gradually until mild tension is felt, and then holding the stretched position six to ten seconds before straightening up. Static stretching is the preferred method of stretching in an exercise program because the chance of injury is less than in dynamic or PNF stretching.

Flexibility Training Considerations

Dynamic, PNF, and Static Stretching Exercises.   Static stretching movements offer several advantages over dynamic stretching movements in developing flexibility. Most sedentary people are likely to have shortened muscles as a result of inactivity and/or failure to use joint mobility to its fullest. Under such conditions, the bouncing or jerking movements associated with dynamic stretching may override or get ahead of the pain receptors' triggering mechanism; as a result, the overstretched muscle will not contract in time to prevent muscle or tendon injury. It is therefore important during dynamic or PNF stretching to use caution against overstretching the muscle. Static stretching, on the other hand, can produce significant increases in flexibility without this potential danger. Accordingly, static stretching is recommended for flexibility improvement.

Specificity of Joint Mobility.   Flexibility is specific. You may possess a high degree of flexibility in some joints of the body and poor flexibility in others. Extensive and prolonged participation in a particular activity will result in development of flexibility only in those joints in which the full range of joint motion is constantly being used while performing the activity.

Factors Influencing Flexibility.   Flexibility is affected by several factors, such as mechanical limitations, activity levels, improper training techniques, posture, and age. Mechanical limitations include such things as natural or unnatural bone formation, fat deposits, and muscle mass, which set definite limits on the range of motion in some joints. Unnatural bone formations include calcium deposits and bone spurs. Also, in heavily muscled or obese individuals it is possible for flexion of the elbow and knee to be limited by the massive bulk of intervening muscle or fat tissue.

People who are physically inactive generally tend to be less flexible than active people. This is due in part to the fact that not only muscles but also connective tissue such as tendons and ligaments tend to shorten through disuse.

Progressive resistance exercises, such as weight training, are sometimes blamed for decreases in flexibility. However, this is a false assertion. Muscle boundness, the term for individuals with bulging muscles and a lack of flexibility, is caused by poor training techniques. In order to avoid muscle boundness, you should perform exercises through the full range of motion, exercise the antagonist (opposite) muscle group, and include stretching in your warm-up and cool-down routines.

Faulty posture can also influence flexibility by causing some muscles to shorten. For example, if you constantly assume a round-shouldered, slouched posture, gradual shortening of the pectoral muscles of the chest will occur. This, in turn, will adversely affect shoulder flexibility.

Age and sex are other factors influencing flexibility. As children develop, they tend to increase in flexibility until adolescence. During the adolescent years, a gradual loss of joint flexibility begins that continues throughout adult life. This decrease can be reduced by a proper flexibility program.

Flexibility and Low Back Pain.   Millions of Americans suffer from chronic low back pain due primarily to weak abdominal and hip flexor muscles in conjunction with poor flexibility of the lower back and hip extensor muscles. The weak abdominal muscles are unable to exert sufficient tension to prevent the pelvis from tilting forward and downward. This causes excessive arching in the lower back and slight displacement of the vertebrae. The resulting pressure on adjacent nerves causes chronic pain in the lower area of the back. You can voluntarily exaggerate the lower back (lumbar) curvature by tilting the pelvis forward and downward to experience similar discomfort.

The solution to this problem of low back pain lies in developing and then maintaining adequate abdominal and hip flexor strength combined with increased flexibility of the lower back and the hip extensors (gluteus maximus and hamstrings). Prompt medical attention is prescribed when more serious causes of back pain are suspected. These include arthritis, kidney disease and spinal defects. Chapter 5 will give additional information on strengthening the abdominals and hip flexors.

The sit and reach test is often used to measure the flexibility of the lower back and hip extensors. This test consists of sitting on the floor with the legs together and extended so that the soles of the feet are flat against the side of the box with the buttocks, spine, and back of the head against the wall, as shown in figure 3.3. Your arms should be extended and your shoulders rounded while your partner slides the yardstick forward or backward to adjust the end of the yardstick with the tip of your fingers. With the yardstick secure in the adjusted position, bend at the waist and slowly slide your fingers along the yardstick as far as possible as shown in figure 3.4 using static stretching. Your partner will read your score to the nearest quarter inch on the yardstick. Norms for college students, ages 17 to 25, are listed in table 3.1.

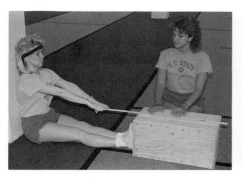

FIGURE 3.3

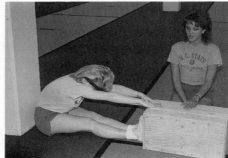

FIGURE 3.4

Flexibility Training Guidelines

The following guidelines should be followed when participating in a flexibility program:

1. Begin the flexibility routine with an easy whole body activity to raise body temperature. This can be accomplished by rope skipping, running in place, or other cardiorespiratory activities. It is generally believed that elevating body temperature through exercise tends to increase the pliability of connective tissue such as tendons and thus provides a greater potential for increased flexibility and less chance of injury.

2. You should never hyperextend, or hyperflex, or lock any joint during the stretching exercise. Do not force body parts beyond their range of motion. Be especially careful during dynamic and PNF stretching where this can easily occur.

3. A minimum of five stretch repetitions should be performed for each exercise. Static stretch repetitions should be held in the stretch position for six to ten seconds and the PNF stretch should be held for four to five seconds. You should be very careful when

TABLE 3.1   Norms for the Sit & Reach.

Percentile	Females	Males
99	21.5	21.5
95	19.0	19.25
90	18.0	18.0
85	17.5	17.25
80	17.0	17.0
75	16.5	16.5
70	16.0	16.0
65	15.5	15.5
60	15.0	15.0
55	14.5	14.5
50	14.25	14.25
45	14.0	14.0
40	13.5	13.75
35	13.25	13.25
30	13.0	13.0
25	12.0	12.0
20	11.5	11.5
15	11.0	10.75
10	10.0	9.75
05	8.0	9.0

Based upon data collected March, 1986 at North Carolina State University. Sample size was 362 females and 442 males.

performing stretching exercises involving the spinal column. Avoid extreme movements of the trunk and neck.

4. Remember, flexibility is specific to each joint. Therefore, stretching exercises must be performed for each muscle group or joint in which increased flexibility is desired.

5. Exercises that do not create **stretch demand**—that is, muscle lengthening beyond normal—will not improve flexibility.

6. Stretching exercises must be performed regularly. The fitness adage, *use it or lose it,* applies as much to flexibility as it does to other components of fitness.

Stretching Exercises

This section discusses a number of stretching exercises. Any of the three methods of stretching can be utilized with these exercises to develop a personal stretching program.

SHOULDER AND BACK STRETCHES

Purpose: To stretch shoulder, chest and upper back.

Starting position (figure 3.5): Arms extended overhead and palms together.

Movement: Stretch arms upward and slightly backwards. Breathe in as you stretch upward, holding the stretch six to ten seconds.

Starting position (figure 3.6): Right arm across chest, left hand supporting right elbow.

Movement: With your left hand, gently pull the right elbow toward your left shoulder. Hold stretch for six to ten seconds. Repeat stretch on opposite side.

Starting position (figure 3.7): Arms overhead, elbows bent. Hold the elbow of left arm behind the head with the right hand.

Movement: Gently pull the elbow downward behind the head. Hold stretch for six to ten seconds. Repeat exercise on opposite side.

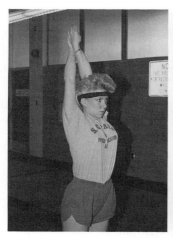
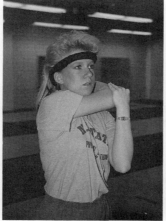
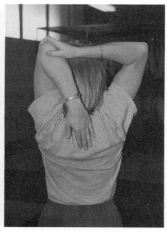

FIGURE 3.5   **FIGURE 3.6**   **FIGURE 3.7**

Purpose: To stretch the latissimus dorsi, a large muscle of the back which extends from the lower spine and attaches to the upper arm.

Starting position (figure 3.8): Right arm diagonally across face, left hand supporting right elbow.

Movement (figure 3.9): With your hand, gently pull the right elbow diagonally across and in front of your face. Hold stretch for six to ten seconds. Repeat stretch on opposite side.

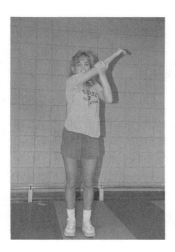

FIGURE 3.8

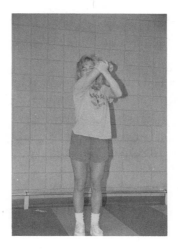

FIGURE 3.9

CHEST AND SHOULDER STRETCH

Purpose: To stretch the chest and front of the shoulder.

Starting position (figure 3.10):   Standing perpendicular to the wall at a distance of approximately six inches to one foot, raise right arm up with elbow bent. Place hand and forearm against the wall.

Movement (figure 3.11):   With hand and forearm placed on wall, rotate body backward around the shoulder joint. Keep hand and forearm stationary on wall during the movement in order to apply the stretch. Repeat sequence on other side.

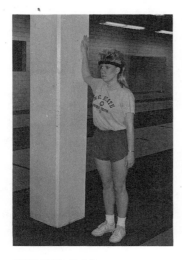

FIGURE 3.10

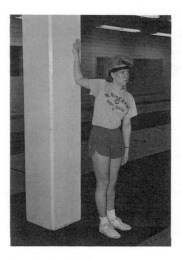

FIGURE 3.11

CHEST AND SHOULDER STRETCH

Purpose: To stretch the chest and front of the shoulder.

Starting position (figure 3.12):   In a standing position, extend both arms at the elbow and move them slightly behind the body at shoulder height. Partner grasps arms just above the wrists.

Movement (figure 3.13):   The partner slowly brings the arms closer together until tightness is felt in your chest and shoulders. The partner then holds the angle and you contract isometrically for five seconds and then relax. Terminate sequence before mild discomfort is felt.

Precaution: This is a PNF stretch and is often used by swim teams. This stretch is contraindicated for many individuals. Remember, always terminate stretching before discomfort is felt.

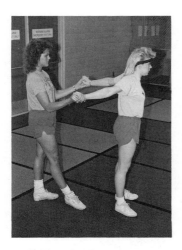

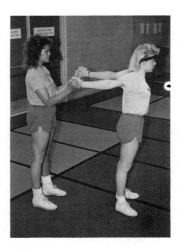

FIGURE 3.12   FIGURE 3.13

SIDE STRETCH

Purpose: To stretch the lateral (side) portions of the trunk.

Starting position (figure 3.14):   Start with your feet approximately shoulder width apart and with your arms raised over your head.

Movement (figure 3.15):   Bend laterally at the waist and lean to one side. Return to the starting position. Repeat the movement to the opposite side.

Precaution: Avoid rotating the trunk as you go through the movement.

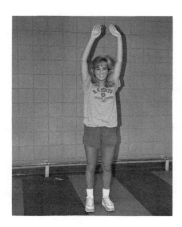

FIGURE 3.14

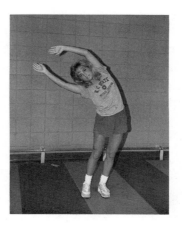

FIGURE 3.15

HIP, THIGH, AND ANKLE STRETCH

Purpose: To stretch the front portions of the hip, upper leg, and lower leg.

Starting position (figure 3.16):   Upright, facing wall, with weight on right foot. The right hand is braced against the wall to maintain balance. Bend left knee and grasp the instep of left foot with left hand. Extend the hip forward to stretch the front of the hip and upper leg. Keep the spine erect.

Movement (figure 3.17):   Slowly pull the left ankle upward and rearward toward left buttock. Hold position and contract by attempting to extend the knee. Hold isometric contraction for four to five seconds. Relax. Slowly move the right foot closer to the hip and attempt to extend the hip forward. Hold position and contract again for four to five seconds. Relax. Terminate sequence before mild discomfort is felt. Repeat exercise on opposite side. Note that this exercise was done using the PNF method.

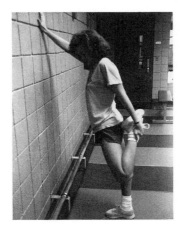

FIGURE 3.16

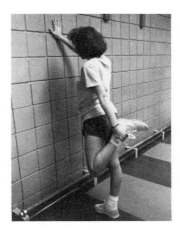

FIGURE 3.17

HAMSTRING STRETCH

Purpose: To stretch the back of the thigh (hamstrings).

Starting position: Seated on floor, feet slightly separated, back of legs flat against floor.

Movement (figure 3.18): Reach forward slowly toward toes. Hold stretch for six to ten seconds.

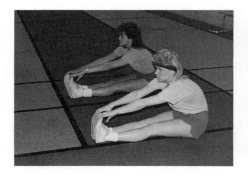 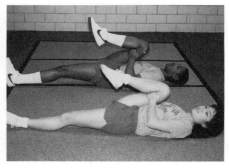

FIGURE 3.18   **FIGURE 3.19**

HIP EXTENSOR STRETCH

Purpose: To stretch the hip extensors (buttocks).

Starting position: Supine, hands at sides, feet together.

Movement (figure 3.19): Slowly draw one knee up toward chest. Grasp hands behind knee and slowly draw knee toward chest. Hold stretch for six to ten seconds. Keep opposite leg flat on mat. Relax and return to starting position. Repeat on opposite side.

INNER THIGH AND GROIN STRETCH

Purpose: To stretch inner thigh and groin area.

Starting position: Stand upright with feet approximately three feet apart.

Movement (figure 3.20): Slide right leg sideways approximately one foot, bend the right knee, and shift body weight toward the right in an attempt to sit over right ankle while keeping the left leg straight. Hold stretch for six to ten seconds. Repeat sequence on opposite side.

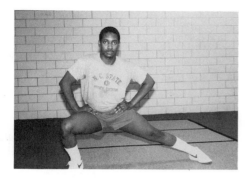

FIGURE 3.20

CALF STRETCH

Purpose: To stretch the back of the lower leg.

Starting position (figure 3.21):   Inclined body position with hands against the wall. The feet are slightly separated and staggered with the near foot approximately 18 inches away from the wall. The near leg is bent at the knee. The heels of both feet are flat on the floor.

Movement (figure 3.22):   Keep body straight in diagonal alignment to the wall. Bend the arms at the elbows allowing the body to lean forward while keeping the heels flat on the floor. Hold stretch for six to ten seconds.

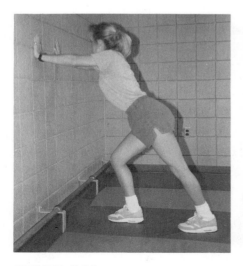

FIGURE 3.21

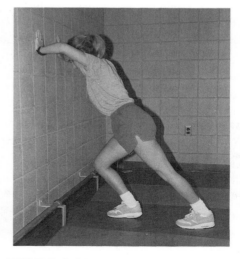

FIGURE 3.22

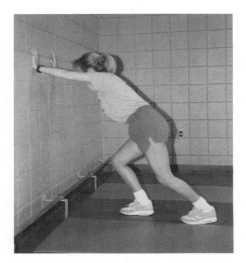

FIGURE 3.23

ACHILLES STRETCH

Purpose: To stretch the achilles tendon.

Starting Position (figure 3.21): Same as for calf stretch. Inclined body position with hands against the wall. The feet are slightly separated and staggered with the front foot approximately 18 inches sway from the wall. The near leg is bent at the knee. The heels of both feet are flat on the floor.

Movement (figure 3.23): Keep body straight in diagonal alignment to the wall. Bend the arms at the elbows allowing the body to lean forward while keeping the heels flat on the floor. Bend the knee of the rear leg. Hold stretch for six to ten seconds.

Remember, flexibility is a component of fitness. Now is the time to incorporate flexibility into your fitness program.

Supplementary Readings

1. American College of Obstretricians and Gynecologists. "Guidelines for Women Who Exercise." Washington, D.C.: ACOG, 1986

2. Chastain, Shanna M. *Aerobics.* Dubuque, IA: Kendall/Hunt, 1988.

3. Corbin, Charles B., et al. *Concepts of Physical Fitness with Laboratories.* Dubuque, IA: Wm. C. Brown, 1988.

4. Cundiff, David E., and Paul Brynteson. *Health Fitness - Guide to a Lifestyle.* Dubuque, IA: Kendall/Hunt, 1984.

5. Devries, Herbert A. *Physiology of Exercise.* Dubuque, IA: Wm. C. Brown, 1986.

6. Hoeger, Werner W. K. *Lifetime Physical Fitness and Wellness.* Englewood, CO: Morton Publishing Company, 1986.

4
Cardiorespiratory Fitness

Cardiorespiratory (CR) fitness is considered by most physical fitness experts to be the most important component of physical fitness. Cardiorespiratory fitness refers to the efficiency of the body in transporting and utilizing oxygen.

The two organs associated with the intake, delivery, and utilization of oxygen are the heart and lungs—hence the term *cardio* (heart) *respiratory* (breathing). Oxygen is the catalyst that initiates the burning of calories to produce energy, a process known as **oxidation.** During exercise, an increase in energy expenditure calls for a similar increase in the amount of oxygen required for oxidation to take place. When your cardiorespiratory system cannot meet the increased demand for oxygen during heightened physical activity, the intensity of the activity must be reduced in order to strike a balance between the amount of oxygen required and the amount that can be delivered.

Since you live in an environment in which the supply of oxygen is unlimited, the problem of obtaining enough oxygen is not an external one, but rather an internal one. The ability of the cardiorespiratory system to process oxygen can be so severely limited in some unconditioned people that even slight increases in energy demands, like climbing a flight of stairs, can cause both heart and respiration rates to rise significantly.

Training Guidelines for Cardiorespiratory Fitness

Certain factors concerning the quality and quantity of training should be considered in the development and maintenance of cardiorespiratory fitness. These include the type, intensity, and duration of exercise. In addition, your physical limitations should be considered.

Type of Exercise. Cardiorespiratory fitness can be attained by participation in a training program in which aerobic activities are used. Aerobic activities are those which are rhythmic in nature, can be sustained for an extended period of time and involve large muscle groups. Aerobic activities include aerobics, jogging, running, swimming, cycling, rowing, speed skating, rope skipping, ultimate frisbee, and many other sustained movement activities.

You should choose enjoyable but vigorous activities that provide a training stimulus. Using a variety of activities in a program tends to reduce injuries caused from overuse, relieve boredom and produce overall fitness.

Intensity.   For healthy young adults the heart rate is a good indicator of the intensity of an activity. The American College of Sports Medicine recommends the intensity of the activity should be vigorous enough to increase the heart rate to 60% to 90% of the **maximum heart rate reserve.** This range is referred to as the **target heart rate zone.** Maximum heart rate reserve represents the percentage of difference between the **resting heart rate (RHR)** and the **maximum heart rate (MHR)** added to the resting heart rate.

Target heart rate lower limit = 60% (MHR − RHR) + RHR

Target heart rate upper limit = 90% (MHR − RHR) + RHR

The best method of determining the maximum heart rate is to have a graded exercise stress test performed on a treadmill. However, due to the expense of the graded exercise stress test, the maximum heart is usually calculated for young, healthy adults by use of a predication formula. An estimate of your maximum heart rate can be computed by deducting your age from 220. For example, if you are 18 years old, 202 would be an estimate of your maximum heart rate (220 − 18 = 202). The maximum heart rate decreases for most individuals at the rate of 1.1 beats per year after the age of 25.

Example: Joe is a 20 year old healthy adult male who has a maximum heart rate of 200 beats per minute **(bpm)** and a resting heart rate of 72 bpm. Therefore, his target heart rate would be:

Lower limit = 60% (200 − 72) + 72 = 148.8 bpm

Upper limit = 90% (200 − 72) + 72 = 187.2 bpm

In order to gain or maintain cardiorespiratory fitness, Joe should monitor his heart rate as he trains and vary the intensity of his activity to ensure that he is within the target heart rate zone.

Figure your target heart rate:

$\qquad$% (MHR − RHR) + RHR = $\qquad$ bpm

Lower limit = 60% ($\qquad$ − $\qquad$) + $\qquad$ = $\qquad$ bpm

Upper limit = 90% ($\qquad$ − $\qquad$) + $\qquad$ = $\qquad$ bpm

You should train near the lower limit of the target heart zone when beginning a program. *Exercise does not have to be unbearable or painful for a reasonable level of cardiorespiratory fitness to be obtained.* Training at the lower limit of the target heart rate zone represents moderately intense activity that can be continued for an extended period of time with little discomfort. Once the benefits of training begin to occur, the training intensity can be safely increased to higher levels within the target heart rate zone.

Duration (Time). The training session should be 15 to 60 minutes of continuous aerobic activity with 20 to 30 minutes being a very reasonable goal. For the greatest gains per unit of time of exercise, thirty minutes appears to be best. Generally, the greater the intensity, the shorter the duration and vice-versa.

Frequency. In order to achieve and maintain cardiorespiratory fitness, you must exercise on a regular basis. Generally, training three to five days per week is recommended. Training less than three days per week appears to be inadequate for gains in cardiorespiratory fitness while training more than five days per week results in a greater incidence of injury. After a desired level of fitness has been reached, it is possible to maintain close to that level by training twice per week. Upon cessation of a training program, a significant reduction in working capacity begins to occur after two weeks.

Weight bearing activities like running and jumping result in a higher incidence of injury than non-weight bearing activities due to the amount of stress generated on the joints of the ankles, knees, and hips. Using a variety of activities in a cardiorespiratory program tends to reduce injuries caused by overuse.

Precautions. It is generally recommended that all individuals over 35 years of age, regardless of health status, complete a physical examination before entering a training program. Also, if you have any medical problems you should have a complete medical exam regardless of your age.

Participation in a fitness program can benefit almost everyone. Once you have identified your physical limitations, you should be able to use the information presented in this textbook to plan a vigorous and enjoyable program which can also be therapeutic.

Before beginning a training session, warm up the muscle groups and joints which will be involved in the workout. Begin the exercise slowly and increase the pace until the target heart rate is reached. Monitor the heart rate periodically to determine if the pace is too fast or slow. After a few training sessions, you will be able to "feel" when the target heart rate is reached. Perform the activity with proper form and technique to reduce the chance of injury and needless fatigue.

Do not overtrain! Initially, the training progression should be slow. If deconditioned and just beginning a program, train every other day. Let the body have the time it needs for recovery by alternating hard and easy days. After the muscles and tendons have toughened and become accustomed to the training routine, the progression can be increased. Remember, using a variety of activities helps prevent injuries from overuse.

Do not attempt to exercise through persistent pain. If localized pain increases during exercise, the workout should be discontinued. If you experience shortness of breath, chest pain, dizziness, or nausea, the exercise should be terminated and a physician should be consulted.

Continue to move at the completion of the training session to prevent the blood from pooling in the working muscles. Monitor the heart to determine the recovery rate during the first couple of minutes after completion of exercise. The rate of recovery will be faster as your fitness level improves. Cool down slowly and stretch at the end of the workout. The muscles are warmest at this time and significant improvement in flexibility can be made.

Assessing Cardiorespiratory Fitness

The most accurate way to assess cardiorespiratory fitness is to measure your oxygen consumption by using a graded exercise stress test on a treadmill. However, since the graded exercise stress test is expensive and time consuming, it is generally not used for most healthy, young adults. More practical, but less accurate tests include the step test and the 1.5 mile run. These measures are often used for determining cardiorespiratory fitness in college fitness classes. Norms for the step test are located in tables 1.1 and 1.2 in Chapter 1. Norms for the 1.5 mile run are in table 4.1.

TABLE 4.1 Norms for the 1.5 mile run for college-age students 17 to 25 years.

Percentile	Males	Females
99	7:21	8:42
90	8:53	11:23
80	9:13	12:00
70	9:27	12:25
60	9:42	12:46
50	10:00	13:14
40	10:16	13:44
30	10:34	14:17
20	10:54	14:38
10	11:30	15:23

Since resting heart rate decreases with improvement of cardiorespiratory fitness, you may wonder why the resting pulse is not commonly used as a measure of fitness. The resting pulse is subject to fluctuations caused by a number of variables including body temperature, environmental temperature and humidity, anxiety and emotional stress, degree of hydration, food intake, and medication. Unless these factors are controlled, resting heart rate as a measure of cardiorespiratory fitness is often unreliable and misleading.

For any given level of fitness, women usually have a higher resting heart rate than men. This is attributable to the fact that women, on the average, have smaller organs. Since the heart and lungs are normally smaller in women, the heart rate and respiration rates must be faster in order to utilize similar amounts of oxygen.

Monitoring Heart Rate

The heart rate can best be monitored at those points on the body where arteries lie close to the surface of the skin. The heart rate or pulse is normally taken at the base of the thumb joint on the inside of the wrist (radial artery pulse) and at the throat just above the collarbone and to either side of the Adam's apple (carotid artery pulse). An important point to remember when monitoring the pulse is not to press too firmly against the artery, especially on the carotid artery. Pressing too firmly will shut off the blood supply.

In counting the pulse rate, the longer the count is taken the more accurate it will be. When measuring the resting heart rate, a long count is desirable. However, a long count will not accurately reflect immediate post-exercise heart rate since the pulse rate begins to drop from the level attained in exercise immediately following cessation of exercise. Therefore, a short count is advisable when taking the immediate post-exercise heart rate. The discrepancy between the immediate post-exercise rate and the rate one or two minutes later can be as much as thirty beats. In order to obtain an immediate post-exercise heart rate indicative of heart rate attained during exercise, a short count started immediately after completion of exercise is necessary. One popular method is to count the heart rate for ten seconds and multiply by six to determine the rate per minute. Another is to count for six seconds and add a zero to the number of beats counted. On the step test pulse recovery used in this textbook, the count is for fifteen seconds. Therefore, the count is multiplied by four to obtain the rate per minute.

Training Effects of a Cardiorespiratory Fitness Program

When the body receives a cardiorespiratory training stimulus on a regular basis, physiological changes begin to occur. The heart enlarges, becomes stronger, and is more efficient. The stroke volume, the amount of blood pumped out of the left ventricle with each beat, increases. The resting pulse decreases as does the pulse rate for any given submaximal workload. Increased capillarization around the cells improves the oxygen diffusion at the cellular level. This enhances the process of replenishing the cells with nutrients and removing metabolic wastes. Also, the collateral circulation feeding the heart is improved. This increases your chances of surviving a heart attack by providing alternate pathways of blood vessels around a blocked artery.

In addition, training enables the arteries to better maintain their elasticity, which enables them to accommodate great pressures. Likewise, the number of red blood cells increases, which provides hemoglobin for transporting oxygen to the cells. Training also reduces low density lipoproteins and increases high density lipoproteins, providing increased protection against coronary heart disease.

Cardiorespiratory Activities

As mentioned earlier in this chapter, cardiorespiratory activities are those activities that are rhythmic in nature, can be sustained for a long period of time, and use large muscle groups in the body. In order to provide a cardiorespiratory training stimulus, these activities must meet the requirements in terms of intensity, duration, and frequency. Hopefully, the activities you choose for inclusion in your training program will be enjoyable. If not, you may experience difficulty in staying with the program. To help monitor your heart rate, use the progression chart in Appendix A.

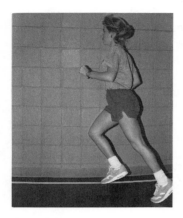

FIGURE 4.1

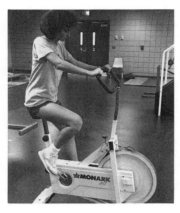

FIGURE 4.2

Jogging and Running.   These activities have become extremely popular in the last fifteen years. They provide an excellent training stimulus for cardiorespiratory gains and are easy to control in regards to intensity, frequency, and duration. Jogging and running require little equipment and give the individual a sense of freedom.

The disadvantage of jogging and running is the high incidence of injuries associated with these activities. Injuries occur for many reasons, including the weight bearing nature of the activities, poor anatomical structure in some individuals, abuse of a proper training progression, and overuse. Common injuries include tendinitis, shin soreness or shin splints, blisters, stress fractures, foot and knee sprains, jogger's nipple, jogger's toe, muscle injuries and strains, chondromalacia patellae (runner's knee), and dehydration. The majority of these injuries could be avoided by proper foot support and clothing, adequate warm-up and cool-down, slow training progression, and staying within the training limitations of your anatomical structure. Research indicates that it is not necessary to run more than three miles five times a week in order to maintain a reasonable level of cardiorespiratory fitness. If you run more than this, you are probably running for a reason other than general cardiorespiratory fitness.

Cycling.   The number of cyclists has greatly increased during the last decade. This trend appears to be partly the result of the increasing popularity of triathalons coupled with the high incidence of running and jogging injuries. Cycling is enjoyable and allows you to tour the countryside while receiving an excellent cardiorespiratory training stimulus. Many people use a stationary bicycle (Figure 4.2) during inclement weather or in areas where traffic is hazardous.

The disadvantages of cycling include dogs, accidents, and the cost of cycling equipment. A common injury in cycling has been chondromalacia patellae, which is a softening of cartilage under the kneecap. However, this injury can normally be prevented by supplementing the cycling program with the leg extension exercise with light resistance and moving through the last quarter of the range of motion to full knee extension. This exercise is discussed in more detail in Chapter 5.

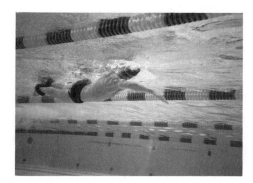

FIGURE 4.3

Swimming.   Swimming is a non-weight bearing cardiorespiratory activity that is excellent when used either as a program in itself or to supplement other activities. Swimming provides a total body workout using the resistance of water. Swimming may be used to maintain cardiorespiratory fitness when resting from a hard workout in another activity or recuperating from an injury. Due to the non-weight bearing and aquatic nature of the activity, swimming offers four advantages over most other activities. First, the cooling effect of the water helps maintain body temperature closer to normal during exercise. Secondly, since swimming is a non-weight bearing activity, there is less trauma to the joints. The third advantage is that blood return to the heart through the veins is faciliated by the effect of gravity being reduced. The last advantage involves the therapeutic nature of the water, in general and in treatment of injuries. In water, you are able to exercise through a full range of motion with minimal resistance, with the buoyancy of the water providing support for the injured limb.

However, swimming also has its disadvantages. Swimming laps in a pool may become boring unless there is variety in your training methods. In addition, eye irritation or injury may occur if goggles are not worn or if the goggles are not adjusted properly. Swimmer's ear can also be a problem if moisture is allowed to remain in your ear canal.

Games.   Game-type activities are very enjoyable and will maintain or improve your cardiorespiratory fitness level if intensity, duration and frequency are sufficient to provide a training stimulus. However, when opponents are not of equal ability, it is sometimes difficult for both or all to receive a training stimulus. Remember, if you use recreational games for a training program, the training stimulus must be provided in regard to intensity, duration, and frequency.

Recreational games used for cardiorespiratory training also have some disadvantages. These types of activities often require you to make quick starts, stops, and turns or cuts. These quick moves provide greater chance of injury to the joints, tendons, and muscles. A good warm-up is very important before recreational games.

Par Course.   Many parks, recreational centers, and even housing developments are now building par courses. A par course consists of several exercise stations located along a jogging trail. Par courses are excellent for improving both cardiorespiratory fitness and muscular endurance. More information concerning par courses is available in Chapter 5.

Interval Training

Slow continuous activity is used to build an aerobic base in a cardiorespiratory training program. Use of these activities permits physiological changes in the body to occur with little chance of injury. In addition, low intensity, long duration exercise produces less soreness in the working muscles than high intensity, short duration exercise.

As your fitness level improves, the desire for competition may increase. The focus of the training program then shifts from maintaining cardiorespiratory fitness to improving performance. The training principles discussed in Chapter 2 now come into play. In order to increase your performance, you must train at a higher level. A popular method of training to increase your speed is called **interval training.** The following factors are controlled in interval training: distance of the interval, time of the interval, type of recovery between intervals, amount of recovery between intervals, and the number of intervals. For example, interval training in running might be to run a distance of 400 meters in a time of 59 seconds. The recovery period may be walking for 45 seconds. This is repeated until ten intervals are completed.

You should adjust your interval training to meet your needs. Interval training is used a couple of times per week by most athletes. Remember to alternate hard and easy workout days. Interval training is a vital method of training when competing in speed and endurance events.

Upon cessation of exercise the heart rate falls, permitting more time for the blood to fill the heart. This results in a strong expansion stimulus being exerted on the heart, which in turn increases stroke volume. Since interval training consists of repeated periods of intense activity interspersed with recovery periods, the repeated attainment of peak stroke volumes stimulates the oxygen transport system more than standard training methods, in which the only recovery period may occur at the end of the workout. Therefore, it is generally agreed that stroke volume is best improved through the use of interval training.

Coronary Heart Disease

A deterioration of cardiorespiratory fitness leads to **coronary heart disease (CHD).** Coronary heart disease is defined as a disease resulting from changes in the arteries supplying the heart and a subsequent interference with blood flow. CHD is the greatest cause of death from disease in the United States today. The results of severe, untreated coronary heart disease include heart attacks and strokes. The likelihood of developing CHD is increased by the presence of one or more of the risk factors listed below. Each of these risk factors can add significantly to the chances of suffering a heart attack or stroke. When several risk factors are combined, the probability of developing CHD becomes even greater.

Risk Factors of Coronary Heart Disease

The American College of Sports Medicine recognizes increased cholesterol levels, cigarette smoking and hypertension as the three most detrimental risk factors for coronary heart disease. Other factors include physical inactivity, improper diet, obesity, personality and stress, age, genetic factors, gender and race.

Cholesterol Levels.　CHD is a multifactorial disease; however, your cholesterol levels appear to be the greatest risk factor. The risk of developing CHD is an exponential function of the total plasma cholesterol. It is generally recommended that your cholesterol level should be below 200 mg/dl. The average cholesterol level of a man who has a heart attack is 244 mg/dl. Although total cholesterol is a strong indicator of possible coronary heart disease, low density lipoprotein (**LDL**) cholesterol is a better indicator and high density lipoprotein (**HDL**) cholesterol, as a negative factor, is yet a better indicator.

Increased levels of HDL appear to offer a protective effect against CHD, for two reasons. First, HDL helps prevent plaque from developing on the walls of the vessels. Second, HDL appears to be capable of picking up excess fats from the blood and transporting them to the liver for elimination.

The best indicator for determining your risk factor for CHD appears to be the ratio of *total cholesterol:HDL*. In a recent study, ninety percent of the individuals whose ratio of total cholesterol:HDL exceeded 6 were found to have significant CHD. However, of the individuals whose ratio was lower than 3.8, ninety percent had no significant CHD. Generally, it is recommended that you be treated to lower your ratio of total cholesterol:HDL if it exceeds 4.5. The treatment normally includes a change in diet and an increase in physical activity. Sometimes medication is prescribed if you are unable to comply with a more vigorous lifestyle and a prudent diet.

Smoking.　It is generally agreed that smoking, especially cigarette smoking, is harmful to health. Cigarette smokers run about one and one half times the risk of CHD as those who do not smoke. When a smoker stops smoking, the risk decreases significantly for development of complications of atherosclerosis. In addition to CHD, smoking is linked to cancer, bronchitis, and emphysema. Furthermore, smoking by pregnant women results in an increased risk of premature births, spontaneous abortions, and stillbirths.

Hypertension.　Hypertension is a term used to describe a condition in which one's blood pressure is chronically elevated. Along with bad cholesterol levels (high LDL and/

or low HDL levels) and smoking, hypertension is one of the most detrimental risk factors for coronary heart disease. If your blood pressure and cholesterol levels are normal and if you do not smoke, your chances of having a heart attack before the age of 65 appears to be less than one in twenty. If you have one of these risk factors, your risk doubles. If you have two of these risk factors, your chances are one in two.

Exercise and Diet. Physical inactivity and an improper diet are contributors to heart disease. Physical activity will have positive effects on both your cholesterol levels and blood pressure. Studies conducted over a 26-year period involving approximately 3,000 subjects have shown that vigorous exercise produces beneficial changes in blood lipids and lipoproteins, which lowers the total cholesterol: HDL ratio. Additionaly, exercise tends to lower the blood pressure in individuals suffering from mild or moderate hypertension.

Diet can also effect both cholesterol levels and blood pressure. Your total cholesterol: HDL ratio can be lowered by adjusting your diet to contain foods low in saturated (animal) fats and emphasizing vegetables, cereals, lean meats such as fish and foul, and skim milk. Generally blood pressure can be lowered by decreasing your ingestion of salt to 5 grams per day. Chapter 6 provides more information on diet.

Obesity. Obesity is often listed as a risk factor of CHD since many obese people also suffer from high blood pressure, which places unnecessary strain on the heart and blood vessels. Most individuals are able to control their weight through diet and vigorous exercise. Chapter 7 provides more information on obesity and weight control.

Personality and Stress. Inability to cope with emotional stress can be a contributing factor to CHD. In contemporary society the drive for peer acceptance and success can force an individual to live and work continually faster, leading to disorders such as gastric ulcers, high blood pressure, and migraine headaches. These physical ills are often indicators of excessive mental stress and a corresponding inability to cope with it. Some studies on personality suggest that certain individuals with overly aggressive tendencies and incessant drives to achieve more in less time are constantly under severe mental stress and tension and are likely candidates for CHD. Their less aggressive counterparts are less likely to experience stress related CHD. Chapter 8 provides more information on stress management.

Age. The incidence of CHD increases with age. Much of this increase can be traced to physiological deterioration attributable to sedentary living rather than to age alone. Longitudinal studies have shown that much of the decline in physical fitness accompanying age can be retarded through regular physical activity.

Genetic Factors. Heredity plays an important role in the development of CHD. This is especially true in cases where there is a family history of high blood pressure, high blood fat levels, or diabetes. Some speculation exists, however, that such relationships may be as much environmental as genetic in nature; that life styles and health habits of offspring often parallel those of their parents or other adult role models. For example, hypertense parents often foster hypertense children; and overfat, inactive parents often have overfat, inactive children.

Gender and Race.   Marked differences exist in the incidences of CHD regarding gender and race. Between the ages of 35 and 44 the death rate of white American males is six times greater than that of white American females. After menopause the incidence of CHD for white females nearly approximates that of white males of comparable age. It is believed that the female's diminished hormone production at menopause is responsible for the increased coronary disease rate.

In the case of race, black Americans appear to be more susceptible to CHD than white Americans. This is true for both males and females. However, in the black American population, both sexes display similar incidence rates.

Although coronary heart disease remains the leading cause of death in the United States, recent health statistics indicate an encouraging downward trend in the death rate from this cause. Most experts believe this turnabout is the result of Americans changing their life styles to include a prudent diet, more exercise, less smoking and better control of high blood pressure.

Misconceptions

There are many misconceptions regarding exercise. Two of these misconceptions relate to head-tilt devices and the wearing of rubber and plastic suits.

Gravity Inversion Devices.   Many fitness facilities have recently introduced gravity inversion devices into their clubs so their members can hang upside down. These devices are supposed to increase flexibility, retard the aging process, reduce blood pressure, improve circulation, relieve back pain, and provide relaxation. Some facilities also recommend performing exercises while inverted on these devices. The physiological effects of head-down tilts of sixty degrees or less below the horizontal are well documented. However, there is little research available on head-down tilts of 180 degrees. A recent study indicates that head-tilts of 180 degrees significantly increased the blood pressure in normal young adults. Therefore, it may be dangerous for hypertensive or borderline hypertensive individuals to use inversion devices. In addition, since blood pressure increases with exercise, you should not exercise on gravity inversion devices until further research is completed.

Rubber and Plastic Suits.   You should not attempt to lose weight by exercising in rubber or plastic suits. This is a dangerous and ineffective practice. Wearing a rubber or plastic suit elevates your body temperature and can cause heat exhaustion. Also, the weight lost from this practice is water weight, which is regained when you relieve thirst by consuming fluids after the workout. Do not wear rubber and plastic suits when exercising.

Supplementary Readings

1. Brown, A. M., and D. W. Stubbs. *Medical Physiology.* New York: John Wiley & Sons, 1983.

2. Castelli, W. P. "Epidemiology of Coronary Heart Disease: The Framingham Study." *The American Journal of Medical Sciences,* Vol. 20, 1983.

3. Chastain, Shanna M. *Aerobics.* Dubuque, IA: Kendall/Hunt, 1988.

4. Cooper, K. "If You are Running More Than 3 Miles, 5 Times a Week. . . ." *Inside Aerobics,* 1984.

5. Friedman, M., and R. H. Roseman. *Type A Behavior and Your Heart.* Greenwich, CT: Fawcett Publications, 1974.

6. Hollman, W., et al. "The Importance of Sport and Physical Training in Preventive Cardiology." *The Journal of Sports Medicine and Physical Fitness,* Vol. 20, No. 1, March 1980.

7. Lemarr, J. D. "Cardiorespiratory Responses to Inversion." *The Physician and Sports Medicine,* Vol. 11, No. 11, November 1983.

8. Marley, W. P. *Health and Physical Fitness.* Dubuque, IA: Wm C. Brown, 1988.

9. Rosato, Frank. *Jogging.* Englewood, CO: Morton Publishing Company, 1988.

10. Schwartz, C. C., et al. "Preferential Utilization of Free Cholesterol from High Density Lipoproteins for Biliary Cholesterol Secretion in Man." *Science,* 200:62, 1978.

11. Segrest, J. P., et al. "Coronary Heart Disease Risk: Assessment by Plasma Lipoprotein Profiles." *The Alabama Journal of Medical Sciences,* Vol. 20, 1983.

12. Tidus, P. M. and C. P. Ianuzzo. "Effects of Intensity and Duration of Muscular Exercise on Delayed Soreness and Serum Enzyme Activities." *Medicine and Science in Sports and Exercise,* Vol. 15, No. 6, 1983.

13. Vu Tran, C., et al. "The Effect of Exercise on Blood Lipids and Lipoproteins: A Meta-Analysis of Studies." *Medicine and Science in Sports and Exercise,* Vol. 15, No. 5, 1983.

14. Zampogna, A., et al. "Relationship Between Lipids and Occlusive Artery Disease." *Archives of Internal Medicine.* 140:1067, 1980.

5
Muscular Strength and Endurance

This chapter deals with the development of muscular strength and endurance. Strength is defined as the maximum force that a muscle or muscle group can exert against resistance during a single effort. Endurance is the ability of a muscle or muscle group to exert force for an extended period of time. Benefits from a strength and endurance training program include increased muscle mass and strength, improved posture and vitality, and a positive self-image. Furthermore, research in weight control indicates that decreases in metabolism, found in individuals as they age, are primarily caused by a decrease in muscle mass. Therefore, continuing in a strength and endurance training program will aid in the battle against creeping obesity, which is discussed in Chapter 7.

Types of Muscular Contraction

The normal response of a muscle fiber to a training stimulus is the development of force directed longitudinally. The amount of force developed by the muscle compared to the opposing force determines the type of muscular contraction.

Concentric Contraction. If the force developed by the muscle is greater than the opposing force, the muscle shortens and thus performs work. This type of contraction where the muscle shortens is called a concentric contraction.

Isometric Contraction. If the force developed by the muscle balances the opposing force, the muscle does not shorten but remains at a constant length. This type of contraction is referred to as an isometric contraction.

Eccentric Contraction. If the force developed by the muscle is less than the opposing force, the muscle lengthens. This type of contraction is referred to as an eccentric contraction.

Skeletal Movement and Muscle Actions

Voluntary movement of your skeletal system is brought about by the shortening of skeletal muscles. There are over 400 skeletal muscles in your body. These muscles are attached to the bones via tendons. In order for skeletal movement to occur, it is necessary that a muscle be attached to at least two different bones. Normally, each muscle acting upon a joint is matched by another muscle called an **antagonist,** which has an opposite action. For example, the biceps brachii (an elbow flexor) and the triceps brachii (an elbow extensor) are antagonists at the elbow. Most movements require the combined action of a number of muscles. Those muscles that act directly to bring about a desired movement are called **prime movers.** Supporting muscles that hold the part of the body being acted upon in the appropriate position are called **fixation** muscles.

Genetic Factors

It is important to realize that genetic factors affect physical performance. These factors include: (1) the number of muscle fibers in a muscle group, (2) the type of muscle fiber that is predominant in the muscle group, and (3) the structure of the muscle fibers in the muscle group.

Number of Muscle Fibers.   Each muscle of the body is composed of groups of muscle bundles that join into a tendon at each end. These bundles are made up of thousands of muscle fibers or cells. In humans, the number of muscle fibers in a muscle group is believed to be established after the embryo has reached the age of four to five months. However, the thickness of the fiber can be altered with training.

Types of Muscle Fibers.   There are two main types of fibers in the skeletal muscle: fast twitch and slow twitch. The muscles of the body consist of a combination of these two major fiber types. The proportion of fast twitch fibers ranges from about 5% to 90% of the total. The higher the proportion of fast twitch fibers, the faster the whole muscle contracts.

Muscles having predominately slow twitch fibers are used for prolonged performance of work. These slow twitch fibers are generally smaller, are surrounded by more blood capillaries, and have more mitochondria (which are responsible for the conversion of food to useful energy) than the fast twitch fibers. The mitochondria are sometimes called the **powerhouse** of the muscle cell due to the fact that adenosine triphosphate (ATP) (the energy source required for muscular activity) is formed there. Slow twitch fibers also have a large amount of myoglobin, which gives a red tint to the fiber. Due to this red tint, slow twitch fibers are sometimes referred to as red fibers and fast twitch as white fibers. Myoglobin is a substance similar to the hemoglobin in red blood cells and can combine with and store oxygen inside the muscle cell unit until needed by the mitochondria.

Fast twitch fibers normally allow a very rapid release of calcium ions and re-uptake of the calcium ions so that the contraction occurs quickly. Individuals with predominately fast twitch fibers are normally better suited for speed or explosive type activities while individuals with predominately slow twitch fibers are better suited for endurance type activities.

Structure of Muscle Fibers.   There are two major types of fiber structures in your skeletal muscle: **fusiform** and **pennate.** The fusiform muscle fibers run longitudinally to and somewhat parallel to the muscle's long axis. A single fiber does not run the entire length of the muscle, but the many fibers that make up the muscle are aligned as a group with the muscle's long axis. The pennate muscle fibers run obliquely to the muscle's longitudinal axis but have tendons that run parallel with the muscle's long axis.

The fusiform or longitudinal fibers are longer and can shorten a greater effective distance than the pennate or oblique fibers; therefore the fusiform can pull the bones through a greater range of motion. However, there are fewer fusiform or longitudinal fibers per unit of area than there are pennate or oblique fibers. Thus, the fusiform fibers can pull the bones through greater range of motion but the pennate fibers are capable of generating more force. The proportion of fusiform to pennate fibers in the muscle determines the range of motion and the amount of force that the muscle is capable of producing.

These are just a few of the genetic factors affecting human performance. Heredity definitely plays an important role and establishes the upper limit in human performance. However, it should be noted that few individuals reach the state of training in which they begin to approach their potential.

Gender

The sex hormone level affects the capacity for muscular size development. The popular myth that exercise, especially resistance exercise, tends to masculinize the physical appearance of women has no basis for most women. The muscle fibers of both sexes are similar, both histochemically and in their distribution. However, females have a smaller cross-sectional area in all fiber types than males. Higher levels of androgens in males account for much of the muscle hypertrophy and strength differences between the sexes. Since women have lower levels of androgens, it is very unlikely that they will obtain the muscle size and strength of men. Women and older men, with lower levels of androgens, apparently gain strength by improving their ability to recruit additional motor units rather than significantly altering the contractile structures of the muscles.

Progressive Resistance Exercise

In Chapter 2 the overload principle was discussed. This principle states that in order for a muscle cell to increase in size and strength, the workload must be increased beyond what it normally experiences. Muscles adapt to the workload placed upon them. When this adaptation takes place, a greater workload must be placed on the muscle for further gains to take place. Progressively increasing the stress (workload) placed on the muscle as adaptation takes place is referred to as **progressive resistance exercise (PRE).** The three most common forms of progressive resistance exercise are isotonic, isometric, and isokinetic.

Isotonic Training.   Isotonic training, commonly referred to as weight training, is characterized by the exertion of force on movable objects such as barbells, dumbbells, and pulley weights. It is used extensively in athletic conditioning to develop muscular power (explosive strength), which is a maximum strength output over a very short period of time. In isotonic training a series of exercises selected to involve all the major muscles of the body are performed against varying amounts of resistance. One complete movement of the exercise is called a **repetition,** and a series of these repetitions, performed consecutively, is called an exercise **set.**

Isometric Training.   Isometric training involves non-moving or static muscle contractions performed against immovable objects such as a wall or a doorjamb, or against one's own opposing (antagonistic) muscles. Researchers have found that static contraction of muscles at two thirds of maximum effort for six seconds can increase strength. Such strength increases, however, are related directly to the specific joint angle at which the isometric contraction occurs. For example, if you repeatedly performed isometric arm contractions with the elbow bent at 90 degrees, maximum strength gains will be at that angle but gains will be less at other angles through the range of motion.

Isometric exercises have some advantages over other forms of resistance exercises: no special equipment is required, little space is needed, and isometrics can be performed almost anywhere. As is true with isotonic exercises, isometrics are often employed in physical therapy programs to rehabilitate weakened muscles associated with injury or disease.

Isokinetic Training.   A muscular contraction is isokinetic when the speed of the contraction is kept constant against a variable resistance. Isokinetic training makes use of a specialized apparatus that provides variable resistance directly proportional to the amount of muscular force being applied by the exerciser, and controls and holds the speed of movement constant during the exercise. This permits a muscle or a group of muscles to encounter maximum resistance throughout a complete range of motion. This accommodating resistance allows more muscular work to be performed and reduces the likelihood of muscle strain, which can occur when attempting to overcome a **sticking point** during isotonic training or when trying to move an immovable object in isometric training. The Nautilus system, although it provides maximum resistance throughout the range of motion, is not a true isokinetic process because it allows for unrestricted speed of movement. It is, however, an effective and popular means of developing strength.

Once in a weight training program, you can expect some improvement in strength in four to six weeks. The rate and extent of improvement is influenced mainly by two factors: your starting level of fitness and the intensity and regularity of your workouts. Strength development is limited by genetic factors affecting the quality of muscle tissue and by your personal drive and motivation.

Most, though not all, studies comparing the various forms of resistance exercise have concluded that all three methods described above can produce significant gains in strength in relatively short periods of time. Recent research seems to indicate that the isokinetic form of resistance training is superior to the other methods for strength gains.

Strength Training Guidelines

Warm-up. A warm-up should precede all training activities. It consists of three phases: cardiorespiratory, flexibility, and muscular endurance. A cardiorespiratory activity such as rope skipping or running in place is performed at a moderate rate to elevate the heart rate and body temperature. Flexibility exercises are used to prevent musculoskeletal injuries from occurring. Submaximal muscular endurance activities are then used to prepare the working muscles for the greater stress that will follow in the workout. You should then perform several repetitions of the exercises comprising your workout, with very light resistance for the final phase of the warm-up.

Cool-down. The cool-down following most progressive resistance training programs consists mainly of stretching exercises to help improve the flexibility of the joints. In general, progressive resistance training programs place little demand on the cardiorespiratory system; therefore, little time is needed to allow the heart and lungs to recover. This is not the case for circuit training, which is discussed later in this chapter. The cool-down after circuit training requires time for the cardiorespiratory system to recover in addition to the flexibility phase.

Breathing. In progressive resistance exercise there is a tendency to hold your breath as the fixation muscles attempt to provide a base from which the prime movers can apply leverage. When the breath is held, the pressure within the thoracic cavity increases as the chest compresses from the actions of the working muscles. This can cause a sudden and dramatic rise in blood pressure, which reduces the return of blood to the heart. This is followed by a drop in blood pressure that may cause dizziness or fainting. This series of events is referred to as the *Valsalva Phenomenon* and can be easily prevented by not holding your breath during exercise. The Valsalva Phenomenon is particularly dangerous if you have high blood pressure. The rule to follow regarding breathing during progressive resistance exercise is to *inhale as the chest is expanding and exhale as the chest compresses.*

Lifting Safety. Proper form should always be used when lifting objects. When lifting an object such as a barbell from the floor, begin with the feet comfortably spread and toes pointed ahead. Lower the hips to a squat position by bending the knees. Keep the head up and the back straight. Begin the lifting motion with the legs, not the back.

Exercises that start with a barbell at the chest or shoulders employ a preliminary movement in which the barbell is raised from the floor to the chest or shoulders in one uninterrupted movement known as a **clean.** The starting position for the clean is the squat position described above. The movement involves a forceful straightening of your legs followed by an upward pull of the bar with the arms. After inertia is overcome and the barbell is rising, the knees are bent slightly and a small step forward is taken to assist bringing the barbell to the chest. The legs are then straightened.

When lifting heavy barbells in the squat, bench press, or overhead lifts, you should always have one or more spotters standing by to assist in removing the weight should you lose control. When using adjustable barbells and dumbbells, always check to make sure that collars holding the weight plates in place are properly fastened to prevent them from sliding off the bar. With machines, check cables for premature wearing and make sure that the weight adjusting pin is securely in place.

Form.   It is important that exercises are performed with good form to avoid injury.

In order to maximize work output, weight training exercises should be performed slowly and deliberately. During the **concentric** phase of an exercise when working muscles are contracting (the *up* movement of the barbell), care should be taken not to swing or jerk the barbell upward. Likewise, during the **eccentric** phase when working muscles are stretching (the *down* movement of the barbell), you should strive to maintain steady tension on the working muscles by lowering the weight slowly and not allowing the force of gravity to do the work.

The term **muscle boundness** implies decreased flexibility, speed of movement, and co-ordination. The notion that progressive resistance training causes this condition is unfounded. Weight trainers who have achieved international recognition for their muscular development or for competitive weight lifting ability have been found to possess above average joint flexibility and speed of movement. However, a decrease in joint mobility will result if you consistently fail to perform weight training exercises through the full range of motion, do not use flexibility exercises, and fail to strengthen the antagonist muscle groups. The one exception to performing exercises through their full range of motion is the squat exercise. Because of the structure of the knee joint, ligament injury can occur to this joint in the deep squat (completely flexed) position.

Selection and Sequence of Exercises.   Total body development is necessary to ensure symmetrical muscular development and prevent loss of joint mobility. Exercises should be selected that will strengthen all of the major muscle groups of the body. Also it is important to avoid the pitfall of constantly using the same exercises in your workout. You will find that you will increase overall strength of each muscle group by slightly varying some of the exercises in your workout program on a periodic basis. This will allow additional muscle fibers in the muscle group to be recruited and thus result in greater overall development.

The sequence for exercising should progress from large to small muscle groups. Those exercises that develop the large muscle groups of the body—squats, cleans, and presses—should form the basis of your program. The amount of time you have for training will influence the exercises you choose for your workout. If your time is limited, your workout should comprise exercises that develop large muscle groups. These exercises will usually develop smaller muscle groups in addition to the large muscles. For example, the bench press develops the anterior deltoids and triceps in addition to the large pectoral muscles. Exercises that develop the smaller muscle groups should be added as time permits. Appendix B provides a workout log for you to record your progressive resistance exercise workouts.

Frequency, Intensity and Duration.   The rate of improvement in muscular strength and endurance is dependent upon the frequency, intensity, and duration of training. Generally, training sessions should be on alternate days, three times per week.

The amount of resistance used in an exercise is determined by trial and error. When beginning a program, you should be conservative regarding the starting resistance for each exercise. After proper form is developed, then increase the resistance as desired.

A resistance that represents 60% to 80% of a muscle's maximum strength is sufficient to produce increases in strength. Generally, such a workload permits the completion of seven to ten repetitions. If you are just beginning a program, you should perform all exercises with workloads that permit the performance of a single set of seven to ten repetitions. After the first couple of weeks, this may be increased to two sets of seven to ten repetitions. When skill and strength improvement permit more than ten repetitions to be correctly performed under maximal (overload) conditions, the resistance should be increased five to ten pounds for succeeding workouts.

Weight Training

Weight training is the most popular form of progressive resistance training. The variety of training systems used in weight training can be geared to your specific needs, priorities, and preferences.

Progressive.   This system is recommended for individuals beginning a training program. The number of repetitions is kept constant but the resistance is increased as gains in strength are made.

Light and Heavy.   In this system, three to five sets are normally performed. Perform the first set against the maximum resistance, which allows five to eight repetitions. On each succeeding set, increase resistance, which will cause the number of repetitions to decrease. Continue until only one repetition can be performed.

Pyramid.   This system is similar to light and heavy except after reaching the one repetition plateau, the procedure is reversed and you work back down the resistance scale.

Super-Set.   A super-set is the performance of a set for one muscle group immediately followed by a set for its antagonist. An example is alternating a set of upright curls for the biceps and a set of tricep presses for the triceps. A multiple super-set would be simply repeating the paired exercises for two or more exercise sets.

Multiple Sets.   In this system you attempt to perform a series of sets using the same resistance and the same number of repetitions. Normally, the number of repetitions will decrease with each succeeding set due to fatigue.

MAJOR MUSCLE GROUPS OF THE BODY

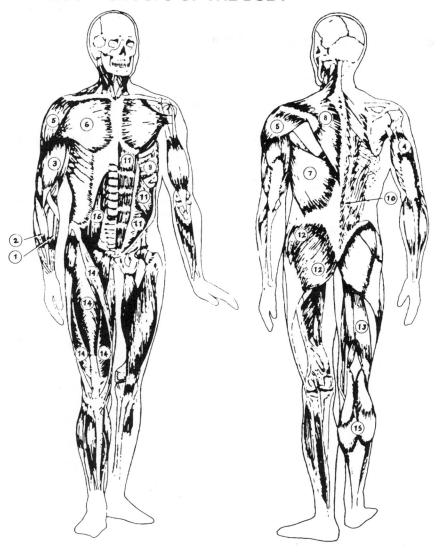

1. Forearm flexors
2. Brachioradialis
3. Biceps
4. Triceps
5. Deltoid
6. Pectoral muscles
7. Latissimus dorsi
8. Trapezius
9. Serratus anterior
10. Erector spinae (spinal extensors)

11. Abdominal muscles
    a. Internal and external obliques
    b. Rectus abdominis
    c. Transversalis
12. Gluteal muscles
13. Hamstrings
14. Quadriceps muscles
15. Gastrocnemius, soleus muscles
16. Iliopsoas (under abdominal muscles)

Adapted from *Muscle Action Chart Number 10* by V. F. Krumdick and Cramer Products, Inc.

Blitz.   If you find that you do not have enough time to train as long as you desire each training session, you can divide your workout training period into smaller units of time but train more days each week. For example, a three hour workout session of 30 or more exercises may be divided into three different and distinct workouts of ten exercises each. Monday's workout may consist of arm and shoulder exercises, Tuesday's workout may consist of chest and back exercises, and Wednesday's workout may consist of leg and abdominal exercises. The progression would be repeated on Thursday, Friday, and Saturday with Sunday being a rest day. Such a program permits the serious weight trainer to lift six days per week but still provides adequate rest for the muscles to recover from the intense workouts.

Strength Training Exercises

BENCH PRESS

Major muscle groups: Pectorals (chest), deltoid (shoulder), tricep (back upper arm).

Starting position (figure 5.1):   Lie in the supine position on the bench with the feet flat on the floor. The barbell is held with a pronated grip (palms facing away) with the hands slightly wider than shoulder width and the arms fully extended above the chest.

Movement (figure 5.2):   Slowly lower the barbell until it touches the chest. Raise the barbell to full extention of the arms to complete one repetition. The head, shoulders, and buttocks should remain in contact with the bench throughout the range of motion of the exercise. The feet are kept flat on the floor.

Precaution: Use spotters. Avoid bouncing the bar off of the chest. **Do not arch your back off the bench as this results in hyperextension of the lower back.** Some individuals prefer to place their feet on the bench instead of the floor to avoid hypertension of the lower back. Be careful, however, when doing this because your base of support is much smaller when your feet are on the bench. With feet on bench, you may experience problems balancing the barbell as you go through the movement.

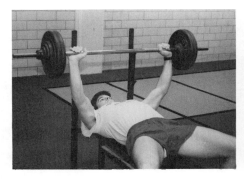

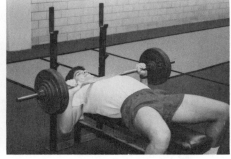

FIGURE 5.1   **FIGURE 5.2**

SUPINE LATERAL DUMBBELL RAISE (FLYS)

Major muscle groups: Pectorals (chest).

Starting position (figure 5.3):   Lie in the supine position on bench with feet flat on floor. Dumbbells are held out from the sides with your palms facing upward and the arms bent at the elbows.

Movement (figure 5.4):   Slowly move the dumbbells upward in an arc by adducting the shoulders. The arc upward is continued until the palms of the hands are facing each other and the arms are fully extended above the chest. To recover, slowly lower the dumbbells along the same plane of movement to the starting position.

Precaution: Avoid using a pressing motion as the dumbbells are raised. **Do not arch your back off the bench as this results in hypertension of the lower back.** You may place your feet on the bench as discussed for the bench press but be sure you are able to maintain your balance as you go through the movement.

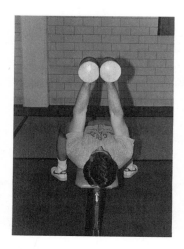

FIGURE 5.3

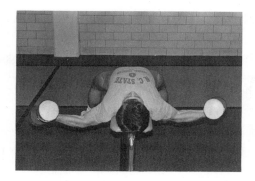

FIGURE 5.4

SEATED OVERHEAD PRESS

Major muscle groups: Deltoids (shoulder), trapezius (upper back), triceps (back upper arm).

Starting position (figure 5.5):   Sit with the feet approximately shoulder width apart. The barbell is in the *clean* position with the hands using a pronated grip. This exercise may also be performed from a seated position on a bench.

Movement (figure 5.6):   Raise the barbell over head to a straight arm position. To recover, slowly lower the barbell to the starting position.

Precaution: Avoid hyperextension or arching of the lower back since it places undue stress on the lumbar vertebrae. Also, excessive bending of the lower back changes the emphasis of the exercise from the shoulder to the chest.

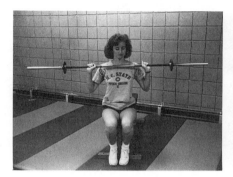
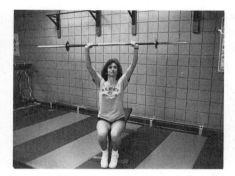

FIGURE 5.5   **FIGURE 5.6**

LAT PULLS

Major muscle groups: Latissimus dorsi (back), biceps (front upper arm).

Starting position (figure 5.7):   Using the lat machine, grasp the bar with a pronated grip with the hands slightly wider than shoulder width. Kneel or sit depending on the length of the cable to the pulley. Hold the bar with the arms fully extended overhead.

Movement (figure 5.8):   Pull the bar down behind the head until it touches the shoulders. To recover, allow the bar to be pulled slowly back to the starting position by the force created by the weight stack, which is attached to the pulley. Avoid leaning the trunk back as the exercise is performed since this changes the emphasis on the exercise to the erector spinal muscle in the lower back.

Precaution: Make sure that the weight stack adjustment pin is secured before beginning the exercise. Avoid contacting the cervical vertebrae as bar is pulled down to the shoulders.

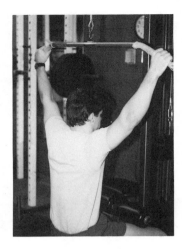

FIGURE 5.7

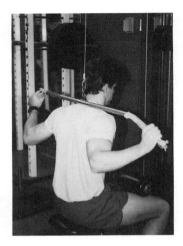

FIGURE 5.8

BENT ROW

Major muscle groups: Rhomboids (upper back), latissimus dorsi (mid back), biceps (front upper arm).

Starting position (figure 5.9): Bend forward at the waist with the trunk parallel to the floor. Flex the knees with the feet approximately shoulder width apart. Using a pronated grip with the hands approximately shoulder width apart, hold the barbell a couple of inches above the floor with the arms fully extended.

Movement (figure 5.10): Keeping the trunk parallel to the floor and knees slightly flexed, raise the barbell until it touches the chest. To recover, lower the barbell to the starting position.

Precaution: Avoid raising the head and trunk. Resting the head on a table top reduces some of the strain on the lower back. However, when using a table top, keep the neck straight to avoid stress on the cervical vertebrae. Don't lift with straightened knees. Keep knees slightly flexed.

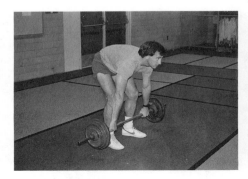

FIGURE 5.9

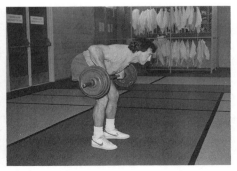

FIGURE 5.10

UPRIGHT ROW

Major muscle groups: Trapezius (upper back), deltoids (shoulder), biceps (front upper arm).

Starting position (figure 5.11):   Stand upright with the feet shoulder width apart and knees slightly flexed. Hold the barbell with a pronated grip with the arms fully extended and the barbell resting across the front of the thighs. The hands are spaced approximately six to eight inches apart.

Movement (figure 5.12):   Raise the barbell until the bar is at chin level. The elbows are held higher than the bar throughout the movement. To recover, slowly lower the barbell to the starting position.

Precaution: Avoid bending backwards. Do not lock or hyperextend the knees during the movement.

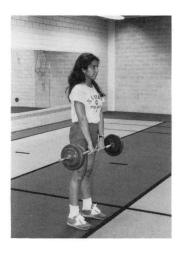

FIGURE 5.11

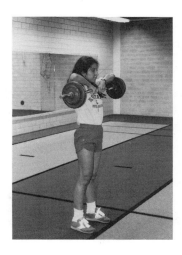

FIGURE 5.12

STANDING TRICEP EXTENSION

Major muscle groups: Triceps (back upper arm).

Starting position (figure 5.13):   Stand upright and hold the lat bar with a pronated grip. Hold the hands approximately eight inches apart and bend the elbows approximately 90 degrees.

Movement (figure 5.14):   With the elbows remaining stationary, press the bar down to full extension of the elbows. Slowly return to the starting position. Except for the forearms the body remains stationary.

Precaution: Avoid leaning forward at the waist.

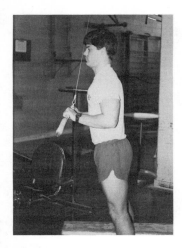

FIGURE 5.13

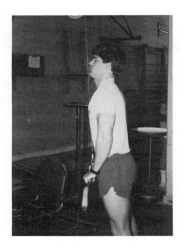

FIGURE 5.14

ARMS: UPRIGHT CURL

Major muscle groups: Biceps and brachials (upper arm).

Starting position (figure 5.15):   Stand with the feet approximately shoulder width apart and hold the barbell with a supinated grip in a straight arm position resting across the front of the thighs. The hands are spaced approximately shoulder width apart.

Movement (figure 5.16):   Raise the barbell forward and upward in an arc towards the chest. The elbows are the center of the arc and should be held stationary at the sides. To recover, slowly return the barbell through the same plane of movement to the starting position.

Precaution: Avoid bending backwards. Do not arch the back. Keep the body in a (strict) straight upright position while doing this exercise. Keep the knees slightly flexed throughout the movement.

LEG EXTENSIONS

Major muscle groups: Quadriceps (front upper leg).

Starting position (figure 5.17):   Sit flat with the padded bar resting just above the ankles on the front of the lower legs.

Movement (figure 5.18):   Extend the knees to the straight leg position (knees are still slightly flexed). To recover, return to a position where the angle of the knee is at least 90 degrees.

Precaution: Do not return to the initial starting position after each repetition as that will place harmful pressure on the knee joint. Return only to the point where the angle of the knee is 90 degrees or greater.

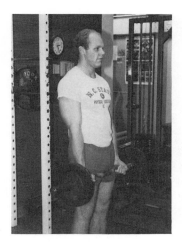

FIGURE 5.15

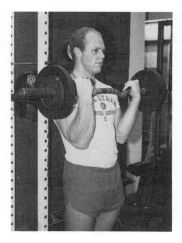

FIGURE 5.16

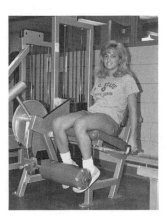

FIGURE 5.17

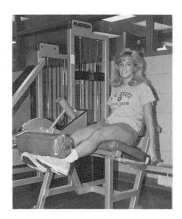

FIGURE 5.18

LEG CURLS

Major muscle groups: Hamstrings (back upper leg).

Starting position (figure 5.19):   Lie in the prone position on the bench with the head down and turned to one side to protect the lower back. The padded bars should rest above the ankles on the back of the lower legs. Hold the handles attached to the bench for support.

Movement (figure 5.20):   Flex the knees to move the padded bars towards the buttocks as far as possible. To recover, return to the starting position.

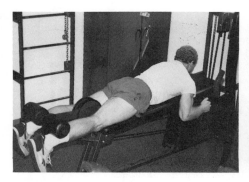

FIGURE 5.19

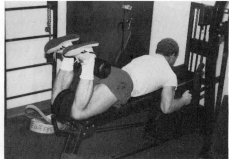

FIGURE 5.20

HEEL RAISE

Major muscle groups: Gastrocnemius and soleus (back lower leg).

Starting position: Stand upright with the feet shoulder width apart. If you are using free weights, the barbell rests across the shoulders, behind the head, and is stabilized by the hands. A block of wood or barbell plate can be placed beneath the balls of the feet and toes to maximize the movement. If you are using the Nautilus multi-exercise machine (figure 5.21), secure the waist strap around the hips.

Movement (figure 5.22):   Slowly raise the heels off the floor so that the weight of the body is supported on the toes and balls of the feet. To recover, slowly lower the heels back to the floor.

Precaution: Keep the body in an upright straight position while doing this exercise. Do not hyperextend the knees between lifts.

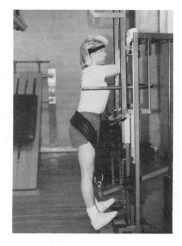

FIGURE 5.21

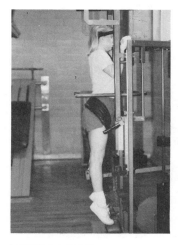

FIGURE 5.22

BACK EXTENSIONS

Major muscle groups: Erector spinae (lower back).

Starting position (figure 5.23): Lie face down across a table or bench with the feet anchored and the torso extending beyond the edge of the bench. Place your hands behind the head.

Movement (figure 5.24): Lift your head and shoulders until they are slightly higher than parallel to the floor. To recover, lower the torso slowly back to the starting position.

Precaution: Avoid fast jerking movements and hyperextension of the back.

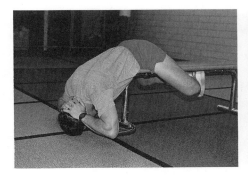 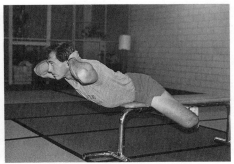

FIGURE 5.23   **FIGURE 5.24**

SHOULDER SHRUGS

Major muscle groups: Trapezius (upper back), deltoids (shoulders).

Starting position (figure 5.25): Stand upright with the feet shoulder width apart, knees slightly flexed. The barbell is held with a pronated grip, the arms fully extended and the barbell resting across the front of the thighs. The hands are spaced a little wider than shoulder width apart.

Movement (figure 5.26): Raise the shoulders towards the ears in a shrugging manner while holding a barbell at waist level. To recover, slowly lower the barbell to the starting position.

Precaution: The lifting and lowering movements should be performed slowly, with the arms straight to provide maximum stress on the upper trapezius muscles.

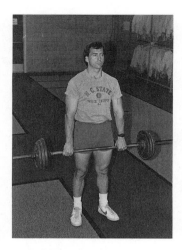

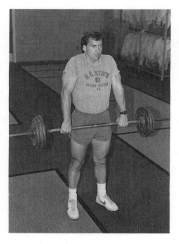

FIGURE 5.25 **FIGURE 5.26**

HALF SQUAT

Major muscle groups: Gluteus maximus (buttocks), quadriceps (front upper leg), hamstrings (back upper leg), erector spinae (lower back).

Starting position (figure 5.27): Stand upright with feet approximately shoulder width apart and toes pointing slightly to the outside. The knees should be slightly flexed. The barbell is resting on the shoulders behind the head. The barbell is held with a pronated grip with the hands slightly wider than shoulder width.

Movement (figure 5.28): While keeping the back straight, lower the body to the half squat position. This position is halfway between the upright position and the full squat position. Keeping the back straight, return to the starting position.

Precaution: If performed incorrectly, this exercise can cause serious back problems. Avoid leaning forward during the movement as this places undue stress on the lower back. Watching a spot high on a wall as the lifter goes through the range of motion often helps keep the back straight. Use light resistance until good form has been developed. Use spotters.

PULL UPS

Major muscle groups: Latissimus dorsi, biceps.

Starting position (figure 5.29): Hang from the pull-up bar with the arms fully extended using a pronated grip (palms facing away). The hands should be slightly wider than shoulder width apart.

Movement (figure 5.30): Without any kicking, swaying or jerking, pull the body upwards until the chin is above the bar and then slowly lower to the starting position.

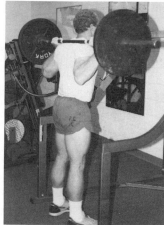

FIGURE 5.27

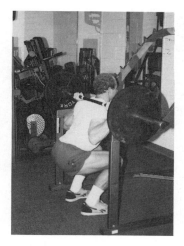

FIGURE 5.28

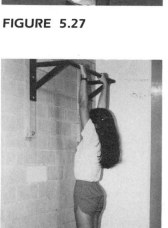

FIGURE 5.29

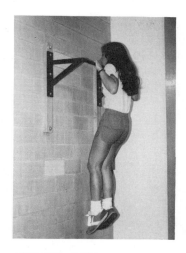

FIGURE 5.30

PUSH UPS

Major muscle groups: Pectorals, anterior deltoid, tricep.

Starting position (figure 5.31):   Lie in the prone position and support the body on the hands and feet with the elbows fully extended. The feet are together, the hands are about shoulder width apart, the back is straight, and the head is down with the eyes looking slightly ahead.

Movement (figure 5.32):   Keeping the body straight, bend the elbows until the chest touches the floor. Return to the starting position.

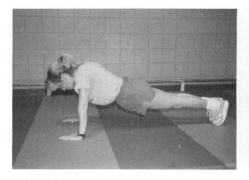

FIGURE 5.31

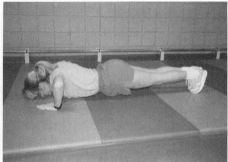

FIGURE 5.32

MODIFIED PUSH UPS

Major muscle groups: Pectorals, anterior deltoid, tricep.

Starting position (figure 5.33):   Lie in the prone position and support the body on the hands and knees with the elbows fully extended. The knees are together, the hands are about shoulder width apart, the back is straight and the head is down with the eyes looking slightly ahead.

Movement (figure 5.34):   Keeping the body straight, bend the elbows until the chest touches the floor. Return to the starting position.

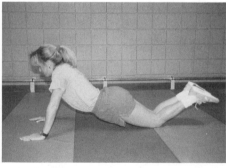

FIGURE 5.33

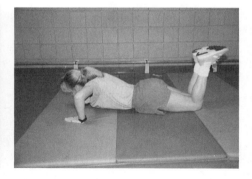

FIGURE 5.34

BENCH DIPS

Major muscle groups: Triceps, anterior deltoid.

Starting position (figure 5.35):   The individual assumes the position portrayed in figure 5.35.

Movement (figure 5.36):   Slowly lower the body down as low as possible and then return to the starting position.

Precaution: Should not be attempted by individuals with poor upper body strength.

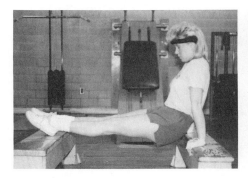 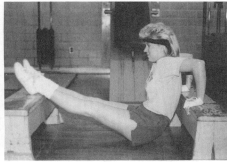

FIGURE 5.35   **FIGURE 5.36**

BENT KNEE SIT-UPS

Major muscle groups: Abdominals.

Starting position (figure 5.37):   Lie in a supine position on the floor with the knees bent at about a 90 degree angle. The feet are flat on the floor and the hands are crossed across the chest.

Movement (figure 5.38):   Flex the trunk until the elbows contact the knees and then return to the starting position.

   Note: If the feet are anchored much of the work is performed by the hip flexors rather than the abdominals.

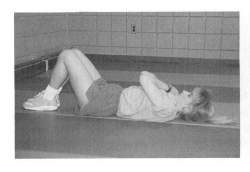 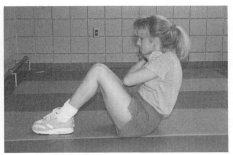

FIGURE 5.37   **FIGURE 5.38**

CURL-UPS

Major muscle groups: Abdominals.

Starting position (figure 5.39):   Lie in a supine position on the floor with the upper legs held perpendicular to the floor. The knees are bent comfortably, the ankles are crossed, and the hands are crossed across the chest.

Movement (figure 5.40):   Keeping the legs stationary, flex the trunk up off the floor as high as possible and then return to the starting position.

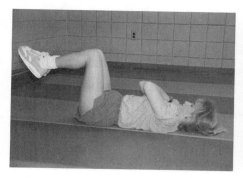 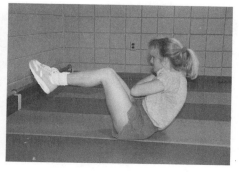

FIGURE 5.39   **FIGURE 5.40**

Circuit Training

Due to the nature of resistance training—that is, short periods of exercise of moderate to intense exertion followed by rest periods—essentially no cardiorespiratory conditioning occurs. Circuit training is a method of exercise that conditions both the muscular and cardiorespiratory systems of the body. The term **circuit** refers to a number of carefully selected exercises, called **stations,** arranged in a circuit and performed in a prescribed sequence. This sequence permits the exerciser to engage in continuous activity by moving from one station to the next without pausing to rest. Progression on a circuit is indicated by decreasing the time required to traverse the entire circuit, increasing the amount of exercise performed at the various stations, or a combination of both.

A distinctive feature of circuit training is its adaptability to a number of situations. For example, a program developed for college age men can easily be modified for other age groups or women. Circuits can be established both indoors and outdoors and can be shortened or lengthened to fit almost any time requirement. If the physical demands of a sport are known, a circuit can be developed that includes skill stations as well as weight training and calisthenic stations. A circuit training program should be intense enough to maintain your heart rate in the target heart rate zone.

An innovation in circuit training is a cross-country circuit training course referred to as a **par course.** A par course consists of several exercise stations located along a jogging trail. As you jog along the trail and arrive at an exercise station, a sign indicates the type of exercise to be performed and the **par,** or number of repetitions, to be performed before jogging to the next exercise station. Typical exercises performed along a par course include push-ups, pull-ups, sit-ups, and a variety of calisthenic type stretching exercises.

Circuit Training Considerations.   In most cases a complete circuit is performed three times. The number of repetitions, amount of resistance used, and speed of performance over the entire circuit determines the workload. Workload, also known as **exercise dosage,** should not be so intense that you are completely exhausted after completing the first lap of the circuit. On the other hand, it must be sufficiently challenging to require performance near maximum capacity during the final lap.

Before you engage in circuit training on a high intensity program, the proper exercise dosage for each station in the circuit should be determined. The recommended method is to spend the first day on the circuit evaluating yourself on each exercise in the circuit. This is accomplished by performing the *maximum* number of repetitions for each exercise in the same order that they appear in the circuit, with a one or two minute rest between exercises. Starting exercise dosage is usually set at *half* the maximum number of repetitions performed. For example, if pull-ups are an exercise in the circuit and you can perform ten, the exercise dosage is set at five.

In setting exercise dosages for muscular endurance exercises such as bent knee sit-ups where 50 or more repetitions are possible, it is best to evaluate maximum performance within a specified time period, usually 30 to 60 seconds. Again, starting exercise dosage is set at *half* the repetitions performed within the time limit. For example, if you can perform 25 sit-ups in 30 seconds you would set the exercise dosage at 12 or 13.

When running is included in a circuit, the minimum time required to traverse a specified distance is *doubled* to set a reasonable exercise dosage. For example, if you are capable of running a quarter mile in one minute set the exercise dosage at two minutes.

Once exercise dosages and total time for completing the circuit are established, you can set new goals as you gain strength and endurance. Generally it is more convenient to keep the completion time constant and to progress by increasing the exercise dosage at the various stations. If barbells are available, weight training exercises can be substituted or added to the circuit. In setting exercise dosages for weight training exercises, the recommended resistance should be approximately *three-quarters* of your ten repetitions maximal load. Thus, if you can upright curl 80 pounds, ten times, you would set the exercise dosage at 60 pounds, ten times.

The following are examples of typical circuit training programs. Program #1 is the least intensive and is basically a calisthenic type exercise circuit. The second program is considerably more intensive and includes calisthenic exercises, running, and weight training.

Circuit Training Program # 1

Station	Exercise	Evaluation	Maximum Perf.	Exercise Dosage
1	Side straddle hops	Maximum in 30 seconds		
2	Push ups	Maximum		
3	Cross-over Curl-ups	Maximum in 30 seconds		
4	Running in place	Maximum steps in 30 sec.		
5	11-ups	Maximum		
6	Alternate toe touches	Maximum in 30 seconds		

Circuit Training Program # 2

Station	Exercise	Evaluation	Maximum Perf.	Exercise Dosage
1	Run/Jog 440 yards	Minimum time		
2	Bent knee sit-ups	Maximum in 30 secs.		
3	Upright curls	Maximum wt. 10 reps.		
4	Run/Jog 440 yards	Minimum time		
5	Prone back lift	Maximum in 30 secs.		
6	Upright press	Maximum wt. 10 reps.		
7	Run/Jog 440 yards	Minimum time		
8	Upright row	Maximum wt. 10 reps.		
9	Half-squat-heel raised	Maximum wt. 15 reps.		
10	Run/Jog 440 yards	Minimum time		
11	Hanging leg raise	Maximum wt. 30 secs.		
12	Supine press	Maximum wt. 10 reps.		

Supplementary Readings

1. Allen, E., R. Byrd, and D. Smith. "Hemodynamic Consequences of Circuit Weight Training." *Research Quarterly,* Vol. 47, No. 3, pp.299–305, 1973.

2. Allsen, P. E., J. M. Harrison, and B. Vance. *Fitness for Life.* Dubuque, IA: Wm. C. Brown, 1989.

3. Corbin, Charles B., et al. *Concepts of Physical Fitness with Laboratories.* Dubuque, IA: Wm. C. Brown, 1988.

4. Darden, E. *The Nautilus Book.* Chicago: Contemporary Books, 1980.

5. Dobbins, B. *High Tech Training.* New York: Simon and Schuster, 1982.

6. Getchell, B. *Physical Fitness: A Way of Life.* New York: John Wiley & Sons, 1979.

7. Gettman, L., L. Calter, and T. Strathman. "Physiologic Changes After 20 Weeks of Isotonic vs. Isokinetic Circuit Training." *Journal of Sports Medicine and Physical Fitness,* Vol. 20, No. 3, 1980.

8. Hesson, James L. *Weight Training.* Englewood, CO: Morton Publishing Company, 1985.

9. Knuttgen, Howard G. "Force, Work, Power and Exercise." *Medicine and Science in Sports,* Vol. 10, No. 3, pp. 227–228, 1978.

10. McDonugh, M., and C. Davies. "Adaptive Responses of Mammalion Skeletal Muscle to Exercise with High Loads." *European Journal of Applied Physiology,* Vol. 52, pp.139–155, 1984.

11. Pipes, Thomas, and J. Wilmore. "Isokinetic vs. Isotonic Strength Training in Adult Men." *Medicine and Science in Sports,* Vol. 7, No. 4, pp. 262–274, 1975.

12. Rasch, P. J. *Weight Training.* Dubuque, IA: Wm. C. Brown, June 1989.

13. Roskamm, H. "Optimum Patterns of Exercise for Healthly Men." *Canadian Medical Association Journal,* Vol. 67, pp. 895–899, 1967.

14. Westcott, W. L. *Strength Fitness.* Newton, MA: Allyn and Bacon, 1983.

6
Nutrition and Health

The complex biological makeup of the human body requires that a proper diet be consumed in order to provide energy, regenerate cells, and maintain physiological homeostatis. "You are what you eat" is taking on new meaning as fast food outlets take in more and more of our food dollars. Some experts believe that the eating habits of the American people have never been worse.

Nutrition has a significant effect on health. It contributes to virtually every function of your body. Nutrients from food are necessary for every heart beat, nerve sensation, and muscle contraction. Good nutrition not only prevents deficiency diseases such as scurvy and anemia, but also improves resistance to infectious diseases and plays a role in the prevention of chronic diseases. Good nutrition is preventive medicine.

The Food Nutrients: What's Available?

There are three categories of "energy" foods: protein, carbohydrates, and fats. Your body utilizes carbohydrates and fats as its main sources of energy. Proteins can be used as energy under extreme circumstances (such as starvation).

Vitamins, minerals, and water are not classified as energy nutrients, but they serve as "catalysts" for vital bodily functions. Water is easily the most essential nutrient for sustaining life.

How Are They Used?

Proteins.   Proteins are complex molecules containing amino acids. They are used in the following manner: (1) cellular growth and repair; (2) enzyme production; (3) energy; (4) blood sugar conversion; and (5) fat conversion. Nine of the twenty-three amino acids cannot be synthesized by the body and must be obtained through the diet; these nine are therefore termed the "essential" amino acids. Although all amino acids function primarily for cellular growth and repair, they can be converted to blood sugar for energy, or they can be converted and stored as fat if the carbohydrate stores are saturated. If used for energy, one gram of protein yields four Calories of energy.

Carbohydrates.   Carbohydrates are your body's primary source of energy. The name *carbohydrates* is derived from the structural components—a pattern of carbon, hydrogen, and oxygen. Carbohydrates can take several different forms, but the basic structure remains the same and includes the following: (1) monosaccharides (simple sugars . . . one molecule); (2) disacchrides (double sugars . . . two molecules); (3) polysaccharides (multiple sugars . . . three + molecules).

The digestive process breaks down polysaccharides and disaccharides into simple sugars for use by the body (figure 6.1). When carbohydrates are broken down and enter the bloodstream, the blood glucose (blood sugar) level is elevated. Your body will use the blood glucose in one of three ways:

1. *Energy production,* if the body needs energy.

2. *Storage as glycogen (glycogenesis),* if liver and muscle is not already saturated with glycogen.

3. *Converted and stored as fat (adipose tissue),* if cells can store no more glycogen.

FIGURE 6.1 Digestive breakdown of carbohydrates.

Enzymes (Saliva) Enzymes (Intestinal)

Complex CHO > > > > Maltose > > > > 2 Glucose Molecules

If one gram of carbohydrate is synthesized and utilized by the body for energy, four Calories will be produced.

Fats. Fats function as a carrier for fat-soluble vitamins, serve as an insulator and body temperature regulator, and can also provide a high amount of energy. A molecule of fat has the identical structural components of the carbohydrate. However, the arrangement of these atoms differ in that the hydrogen count easily exceeds the oxygen count in a fat molecule. Of the two dietary fats, one fatty acid (*saturated*) has a single bond between the carbon atoms. The other (*unsaturated*) has a double bond between the carbon atoms. This difference reduces the unsaturated fatty acid's potential for binding hydrogen (figure 6.2). Unsaturated fats are easier to convert into short-carbon chains than saturated fats. Therefore, it is recommended that unsaturated fats be taken in a 2:1 ratio over saturated fats. High saturated fat diets contribute to atherosclerosis (plaque in arteries).

Fats are initially broken down in the small intestine. Once fat enters the bloodstream, the enzyme lipoprotein lipase converts the fat into fatty acids that are used for energy

FIGURE 6.2 Molecular differences between fats.

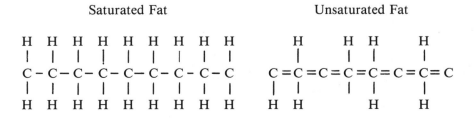

synthesis or stored as triglycerides in adipose tissue. If needed, the stored fat can be removed from the adipose cells and used as energy. One gram of fat will yield nine Calories of energy.

Vitamins.   Vitamins are essential for controlling bodily functions such as regulating metabolic reactions for energy synthesis. Some vitamins (A, D, K, E) are fat-soluble and can be stored in the body. Vitamins C and B are water soluble and must be ingested on a daily basis. See table 6.1 for the functions and sources of each vitamin.

Minerals.   The most valuable function of a mineral is to serve as a regulator of cellular metabolism. Minerals are classified as major and trace minerals. The sources and functions for essential minerals are listed in table 6.2.

Water.   The body contains water in extracellular (outside the cell) and intracellular (inside the cell) areas. Blood, saliva, fluids from glands and the intestine, and fluids excreted from the skin are extracellular areas high in water content. Water is a vital element in bodily function even though it does not actually contribute to the nutritional value of food. Water comprises approximately 60% of body weight and acts as a transfer medium for vital bodily processes. It also aids in body temperature regulation.

The typical adult requires approximately 2.5 liters of water every day. Large quantities of water are excreted as urine and bodily waste while smaller amounts are lost from respiration and cellular metabolism. Water loss from exercise varies from individual to individual. In general, the warmer the environment is, the more an individual will need to perspire in order to aid the body in temperature regulation. Consequently, this elevates the body's need to replenish its water stores. The thirst for water is usually satisfied before the body's stores have been properly replenished. Therefore, we should "force" extra liquids, especially after exercising in the heat (figure 6.3).

FIGURE 6.3   Water balance in man.

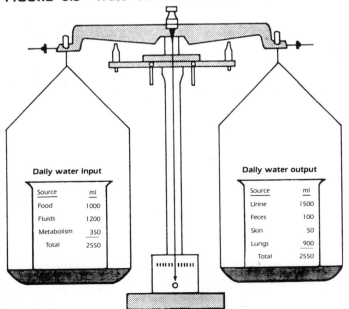

Daily water input	
Source	ml
Food	1000
Fluids	1200
Metabolism	350
Total	2550

Daily water output	
Source	ml
Urine	1500
Feces	100
Skin	50
Lungs	900
Total	2550

Reprinted by permission. From McArdle, Katch, and Katch, *Exercise Physiology: Nutrition and Human Performance.* © 1986, Lea & Febiger, Philadelphia.

TABLE 6.1   Major functions of vitamins.

Nutrient	Good Sources	Major Functions	Deficiency Symptoms
Vitamin A	Milk, cheese, butter, fortified margarine, eggs, liver orange/ yellow/dark green fruits and vegetables	Required for healthy bones, teeth, skin, gums, and hair. Maintenance of inner mucous membranes, thus increasing resistance to infection. Adequate vision in dim light.	Night blindness, decreased growth, decreased resistance to infection, rough-dry skin
Vitamin D	Fortified milk, cod liver oil, salmon, tuna, egg yolk	Necessary for bones and teeth. Needed for calcium and phosphorus absorption.	Rickets (bone softening), fractures and muscle spasms
Vitamin E	Vegetable oils, yellow and green leafy vegetables, margarine, wheat germ, whole grain breads and cereals	Related to oxydation and normal muscle and red blood cell chemistry.	Leg cramps, red blood cell breakdown
Vitamin K	Green leafy vegetables, cauliflower, cabbage, eggs, peas, and potatoes	Essential for normal blood clotting.	Hemorrhaging
Vitamin B$_1$ (Thiamine)	Enriched bread, lean meat, fish, liver, pork, poultry, organ meats, legumes, nuts, dried yeast, and milk	Assists in proper use of carbohydrates. Normal functioning of nervous system. Maintenance of good appetite.	Loss of appetite, nausea, confusion, cardiac abnormalities, muscle spasms
Vitamin B$_2$ (Riboflavine)	Eggs, milk, leafy green vegetables, whole grains, lean meats, dried beans and peas	Contributes to energy release from carbohydrates, fats, and proteins. Needed for normal growth and development, good vision and healthy skin.	Cracking of the corners of the mouth, inflammation of the skin, impaired vision
Vitamin B$_6$ (Pyridoxine)	Vegetables, meats, whole grain cereals, soybeans, peanuts, and potatoes	Necessary for protein and fatty acids metabolism, and normal red blood cell formation.	Depression, irritability, muscle spasms, nausea
Vitamin B$_{12}$	Meat, poultry, fish, liver, organ meats, eggs, shellfish, milk, and cheese	Required for normal growth, red blood cell formation, nervous system and digestive tract functioning.	Impaired balance, weakness, drop in red blood cell count
Niacin	Liver and organ meats, meat, fish, poultry, whole grains, enriched breads, nuts, green leafy vegetables, and dried beans and peas	Contributes to energy release from carbohydrates, fats, and proteins. Normal growth and development, and formation of hormones and nerve-regulating substances.	Confusion, depression, weakness, weight loss
Biotin	Liver, kidney, eggs, yeast, legumes, milk, nuts, dark green vegetables	Essential for carbohydrate metabolism and fatty acid synthesis.	Inflamed skin, muscle pain, depression, weight loss
Folic Acid	Leafy green vegetables, organ meats, whole grains and cereals, and dried beans	Needed for cell growth and reproduction and red blood cell formation.	Decreased resistance to infection
Pantothenic Acid	All natural foods, especially liver, kidney, eggs, nuts, yeast milk, dried peas and beans, and green leafy vegetables	Related to carbohydrate and fat metabolism.	Depression, low blood sugar, leg cramps, nausea, headaches
Vitamin C (Ascorbic Acid)	Fruits and vegetables	Helps protect against infection. Formation of collagenous tissue. Normal blood vessels, teeth and bones.	Slow healing wounds, loose teeth, hemorrhaging, rough-scaly skin, irritability

From *Lifetime Physical Fitness & Wellness: A Personalized Program* by Werner W. K. Hoeger.

TABLE 6.2 *Major functions of minerals.*

Nutrient	Good Sources	Major Functions	Deficiency Symptoms
Calcium	Milk, cheese, green leafy vegetables, dried beans, sardines, salmon, and citrus fruits	Required for strong teeth and bone formation. Maintenance of good muscle tone, heart beat, and nerve function.	Bone pain and fractures, periodontal disease, muscle cramps
Iron	Organ meats, lean meats, seafoods, eggs, dried peas and beans, nuts, whole and enriched grains, and green leafy vegetables	Major component of hemoglobin. Aids in energy utilization.	Nutritional anemia, and overall weakness
Phosphorus	Meats, fish, milk, eggs, dried beans and peas, whole grains, and processed foods	Required for bone and teeth formation. Energy release regulation.	Bone pain and fracture, weight loss, and weakness
Zinc	Milk, meat, seafood, whole grains, nuts, eggs, and dried beans	Essential component of hormones, insulin, and enzymes. Used in normal growth and development.	Loss of appetite, slow healing wounds, and skin problems
Magnesium	Green leafy vegetables, whole grains, nuts, soybeans, seafood, and legumes	Needed for bone growth and maintenance. Carbohydrate and protein utilization. Nerve function. Temperature regulation.	Irregular heartbeat, weakness, muscle spasms, and sleeplessness
Sodium	Table salt, processed foods, and meat	Body fluid regulation. Transmission of nerve impulse. Heart action.	Rarely seen
Potassium	Legumes, whole grains, bananas, orange juice, dried fruits, and potatoes	Heart action. Bone formation and maintenance. Regulation of energy release. Acid-base regulation.	Irregular heartbeat, nausea, weakness

From *Lifetime Physical Fitness & Wellness: A Personalized Program* by Werner W. K. Hoeger.

How Much Do You Need and Where Do You Get It?

Men and women need a certain amount of food to meet their total daily energy requirements. References to Calories are made when you attempt to quantify that energy requirement. A kilocalorie (commonly referred to as Calorie) is the amount of energy needed to heat one liter of water one degree centigrade. The average man needs approximately 2700 calories per day while the average woman requires about 2100 calories.

From the previous section, you should know how the different energy nutrients function. Now you need some idea as to how much of each product is necessary to maintain nutritional fitness, and what foods you should consume to obtain this desirable balance.

Protein. The recommended daily allowance (RDA) of protein for adults is a minimum of .4 grams per kilogram body weight. The ideal intake should be .9 grams per kilogram body weight. For infants and growing children, the RDA is 2.0 and 4.0 grams per kilogram body weight. Protein should constitute 15% to 20% of your daily caloric total.

Proteins that contain the essential amino acids can be consumed from plant and animal cells. *Complete proteins* contain all the essential amino acids in quality and quantity for nitrogen balance, tissue growth, and tissue repair. *Incomplete proteins* lack one or more of the essential amino acids. Quality protein foods (complete proteins) are usually of animal origin, such as eggs, meat, fish, poultry, and milk. However, most complete proteins are high in cholesterol, which increases the risk for coronary heart disease. Lower quality (incomplete) protein sources are mostly of vegetable origin, such as beans, peas, nuts, and breads. Through careful planning it is possible for you to combine a variety of the incomplete protein foods to meet the RDA for all essential amino acids without having to consume foods high in cholesterol.

Carbohydrates. The typical American diet of total calories consists of approximately 45% to 55% carbohydrates. Since the body operates primarily on carbohydrates, this average should be closer to 60% to 70%. The key point to remember is that different kinds of carbohydrates are available, and some provide a better source of nutrients than others. As was mentioned in an earlier section, we ingest three types of carbohydrates daily; they are *monosaccharides, disaccharides,* and *polysaccharides.*

Monosaccharides are simple (one molecule) sugars. They include *glucose, fructose,* and *galactose.* Glucose is also called *dextrose* or *blood sugar.* It is a natural food sugar or can be the end result of complex carbohydrate breakdown. This is the final form in which carbohydrates are used for energy. Fructose is also called *fruit sugar* because it is found in fruits and honey. It is easily converted to glucose. Galactose is not found in food. This simple sugar must be produced from *lactose* (milk sugar).

Disaccharides are double sugars formed from the combination of two monosaccharides. They include *sucrose, lactose,* and *maltose.* Sucrose is also called table sugar. This is the most commonly used sugar in the diet; it occurs mostly in cane and brown sugar (SUCROSE = GLUCOSE + FRUCTOSE). Lactose is also called *milk sugar.* It is found only in milk, but can be artificially produced (LACTOSE = GLUCOSE + GALACTOSE). Maltose occurs in malt products. It is not a large component of the average diet.

Polysaccharides are a combination of three or more simple sugars. There are two forms, plant and animal. The plant polysaccharides are also called *starch* and *cellulose.* The starch component is found in grain products that are used to make pastas, cereals, and breads. Starch is also found in most vegetables. *Cellulose* refers to the structural plant parts that are not readily digested by humans. These fibrous components (i.e., roots, stems, seeds, leaves, fruit coverings) add "bulk" to the diet and aid in "cleansing" the gastrointestinal tract. Animal polysaccharides are also called *glycogen.* This is the muscle and liver storage form for polysaccharides. This carbohydrate can be converted and used as energy, especially during exercise.

Since the body appears to digest complex carbohydrates more slowly and more efficiently than simple sugars, the majority of carbohydrate intake should be in the form of polysaccharides. A diet higher in complex sugars and lower in sucrose can also lessen the insulin response that often occurs after ingesting foods high in refined sugar content. Additionally, the vitamin and mineral contents of carbohydrates in natural form (fruits, vegetables, whole grain products) are much higher than those of the processed sugars. A step in the right direction is for you to determine which foods contain "hidden sugars" (sucrose) and attempt to replace these with complex carbohydrates.

Fats. The typical American diet consists of an unacceptable amount of fat, particularly saturated fat. Many people consume 35% to 40% of their daily calorie total in the form of fats. This is too high. Your body will adapt quite nicely if these percentages are reduced to 15% to 20% with the majority coming in the unsaturated variety. However, the average American may have a difficult time reaching this level simply because of a traditional preference for foods high in fat. A positive step in lowering the saturated fat content of your diet is to identify the high risk foods and attempt to substitute foods lower in fat.

A critical factor in the fat content of many foods involves the preparation. A classic example is fried foods—many nutritious foods are altered by the tendency to fry with animal and vegetable oils that are usually 100% fat.

Some primary sources of fats are red meats, butter, cheese, cream, and peanuts. Table 6.3 lists various sources of saturated and unsaturated fats.

TABLE 6.3 Common sources of fat.

Food	Percent Fat	Percent Saturated	Percent Unsaturated
Animal sources			
Beef	16–42	52	48
Chicken	10–17	30	70
Beef heart	6	50	50
Lamb	19–29	60	40
Ham, sliced	23	45	55
Pork	32	45	55
Veal cutlet	10	50	50
Butter	81	55	36
Plant sources			
Cashew nuts	48	18	82
Peanut butter	50	25	75
Carrots	0	0	0
Potato chips	35	25	75
Margarine	81	26	66
Corn oil	100	7	78
Cottonseed oil	100	21.5	71.5
Olive oil	100	14	86
Soybean oil	100	14	71.5

Reprinted by permission. From McArdle, Katch, and Katch, *Exercise Physiology: Nutrition and Human Performance.* © 1986, Lea & Febiger, Philadelphia.

Since the typical American diet is thought to be inadequate to maintain optimal health and freedom from disease, the Senate Committee on Nutrition and Human Needs endorsed the *Prudent Diet* to assist you in your daily eating habits. This committee, with recommendations from nutrition and food experts, established the following seven dietary goals:

1. To avoid overweightness, balance the caloric intake with the caloric expenditure; if overweight, decrease the caloric intake and increase the caloric expenditure.
2. Increase the consumption of complex carbohydrates and *naturally occuring* sugars.
3. Reduce the consumption of refined and processed sugars.
4. Reduce the total consumption of fats.
5. Reduce saturated fat consumption and balance that with polyunsaturated and monounsaturated fats.
6. Reduce cholesterol consumption to about 300 mg per day.
7. Limit the intake of sodium by reducing the intake of salt to about 5 grams per day.

These suggested changes in your diet are generally thought to be beneficial in reducing the chronic diseases (heart disease, diabetes) that plague modern society. These changes can be made by:

1. Increasing the consumption of fruits, vegetables, and whole grains.
2. Decreasing the consumption of meat and increasing the consumption of poultry and fish.
3. Decreasing the consumption of foods high in fat and partially substituting polyunsaturated fat for saturated fat.
4. Substituting non-fat milk for whole milk.
5. Decreasing the consumption of butterfat, eggs, and other high cholesterol sources.
6. Decreasing the consumption of sugar and foods high in sugar content.
7. Decreasing the consumption of salt and foods high in salt content.

Alcohol

The abstention or prudent use of alcoholic beverages is an individual responsibility. If you decide to drink alcoholic beverages, it is important that you develop a responsible pattern of behavior that can be followed for a lifetime; in addition, you need to understand some basic facts regarding its use.

Alcohol is a depressant and therefore slows the mental and physical functions of the body. These functions include memory recall, cognitive thinking, reaction time, strength, and skills involving fine motor movement patterns. It has been estimated that over 50% of all fatal traffic accidents involve a drinking driver. In addition, alcoholic beverages are high in calories but low in nutrients; this means heavy drinkers often have problems with overfatness and nutrition since they tend to allow alcohol to displace the more nutritious foods in their diets. It is common knowledge that heavy alcohol use causes cirrhosis of the liver. Also, evidence now supports the concept that drinking alcohol during a pregnancy may cause permanent damage to the baby.

When a drinking problem exists, the negative effects rarely harm only you, the drinker. Friends, family members, and others who come into contact with the drinker are also affected.

Your tolerance or lack of tolerance to alcohol can be affected by many things including an empty stomach, mood and attitude, food consumption, illness, physical problems such as diabetes, and the amount and type of beverage consumed. In addition, the faster you drink, the faster the alcohol reaches the bloodstream. Therefore, if you do drink, the beverage should be sipped, not gulped. Finally, the smaller the body weight, the higher the blood alcohol level for a given amount of alcohol consumed.

Information concerning drinking and its related problems is available at most student health and counseling services. Be smart! Don't let alcohol mess up an enjoyable university life.

Commonly Asked Questions in Nutrition

The following are questions concerning diet and fitness.

1. *Why are whole grains better than refined grains?* Trace amounts of minerals, vitamin B, and other nutrients are removed during the refining process. Some of these nutrients are added back during the enrichment process, but whole grains contain more fiber and nutrients than refined grains.

2. When training intensively, should a person increase his or her intake of protein? Yes, but only for the first week. Apparently, the initiation of intensive training program causes individuals on a diet containing "normal" amounts of protein (.9 grams per kilogram of body weight) to go into negative nitrogen balance (net loss of protein). During the first week of training, the protein intake should be increased to 1.5 grams per kilogram of body weight. After the first week, the normal recommended amount of .9 grams per kilogram of body weight appears to be sufficient.

3. *Does sugar consumption in the form of candy or soda before an exercise event provide quick energy?* Sugar consumption before an exercise event results in an insulin reaction; blood sugar (glucose) is removed from the blood, leaving you with less energy than you would have had without the sugar.

4. *Are vitamin and mineral supplements necessary?* The body generally cannot utilize additional quantities of any vitamin other than the amount required for normal function. As long as the diet provides adequate nutrients, supplementation does not help.

5. *Is bread fattening?* No. Bread is not only nutritious (complex carbohydrate, calcium, iron, niacin, riboflavin, thiamine, protein) but is also low in calories (70 calories/slice). Bread becomes fattening when we add butter, margarine, jams, and meats to it, though the bread gets the blame. Please remember that any food taken in excess can be converted and stored as fat.

Supplementary Readings

1. Allsen, Philip E., J. M. Harrison, and B. Vance, *Fitness for Life*. Dubuque, IA: Wm. C. Brown, 1989.

2. Bucher, Charles A., and W. E. Prentice. *Fitness for College and Life*. St. Louis, MO: C. B. Mosby, 1987.

3. Dintiman, G. B., S. E. Stone, J. C. Pennington, R. G. Davis. *Discovering Lifetime Fitness*. St. Louis, MO: West Publishing, 1988.

4. Fox, Edward L. *Lifetime Fitness*. Dubuque, IA: Wm. C. Brown, 1988.

5. McArdle, William D., F. I. Katch, and V. L. Katch. *Energy, Nutrition, and Human Performance*. Philadelphia, PA: Lea and Febiger, 1986.

6. Select Committee on Nutrition and Human Needs, *Dietary Goals for the United States*. U.S. Senate: Washingtin, D.C. Government Printing Office, December, 1977.

7
Weight Control

Thirty to sixty percent of the American public are considered obese. However, obesity should be distinguished from being overweight as indicated by height–weight charts used by insurance companies. Excessive body weight may be due to an accumulation of body fat or muscle mass. For example, muscular men often have body weights that far exceed the norms for their height and weight and yet have a low percentage of body fat. Obesity is being *overfat,* not *overweight.*

The amount of fat accumulation on your body is commonly expressed as a percentage of the total body weight and is referred to as "percent body fat." Table 7.1 can be used to classify body composition based on percent body fat.

TABLE 7.1 *Body composition based on percent body fat.*

| Classification | Percent Body Fat | |
	Men	Women
Very lean	10%	12%
Lean	11–13%	13–17%
Average	14–15%	18–23%
Fat	16–17%	24–27%
Overfat (obese)	≥ 18%	≥ 28%

Assessment of Body Fat

Many methods can be used to estimate your body fat. Less accurate methods include pinching an inch, circumference measurements, and looking in the mirror. Although each of these methods does help, more accurate methods are available. Physiology labs normally use the *hydrostatic* weighing and measurement of body volume method, which is considered by the majority of experts to be most accurate. However, this method is complex, time consuming, space requiring, and expensive. Another method, which correlates very well with hydrostatic weight and measurement of body volume, is the use of *skinfold measures.* Using a set of skinfold calipers, the thickness of the skin is measured at various sites by gently grasping the skin between the thumb and index finger and drawing the skin away from the body. Normally the skinfold is drawn away from the body in the vertical plane; however, if the natural flow of the skin is in a diagonal or horizontal plane, the skinfold is measured in the appropriate natural plane. Table 7.2 lists percent body fat calculations using the sum of skinfold measures taken at the chest, abdomen, and thigh for men. Table 7.3 lists the sum of the measures taken at the triceps, iliac crest, and thigh for women.

Hazards of Obesity

Physical appearance and social acceptance tend to be the dominant reasons that people are concerned with maintaining a normal body weight. Severe emotional and physical problems can occur from being overfat.

Emotional Problems.   Older children and adolescents are especially concerned about appearance and can suffer severe psychological maladjustments as a result of disfigurement caused by obesity. Overfat boys and girls are often subjected to ridicule and social rejection by their unthinking peers. The inferiority complexes and social withdrawals that often result from such non-acceptance can leave emotional scars that may remain with the overfat child throughout life.

Physical Problems.   As serious as the adverse effects of obesity on social and psychological well-being are, the destructive effects of obesity on physical health are even more pronounced. Obesity places an additional burden upon circulation and respiration, making the individual more susceptible to heart, lung, and blood vessel disorders. Overfat individuals have less exercise tolerance, greater difficulty in normal breathing, and a higher frequency of respiratory infections than people with normal body fat levels. Also, overfat individuals possess a higher risk for diabetus mellitus, high blood pressure, high cholesterol, kidney and gall bladder disease, and atherosclerosis. In general, medical statistics indicate the incidence of most diseases is greater in people who are overfat.

Causes of Obesity

Obesity occurs when your average daily caloric intake contains more calories than are needed to maintain body functions and meet the caloric expenditures of daily activities. Excess calories are stored in your body's fat cells in the form of adipose (fat) tissue and gradually increase fat weight to an undesirable amount. If you balance caloric intake with caloric expenditure, body weight stabilizes and further increases in fat storage do not occur. Creating a negative caloric imbalance results in a reduction in body weight as your body "borrows" calories from its fat cells to make up the caloric deficit.

TABLE 7.2*   Percent fat estimates for men using the sum of the chest, abdominal, and thigh skinfolds.**

Male Sum of Skin Folds (mm)	<23	Age 23 to 27	28 to 32	33 to 37	38 to 42	43 to 47	48 to 52	53 to 57	Over 58
8–10	1.3	1.8	2.3	2.9	3.4	3.9	4.5	5.0	5.5
11–13	2.2	2.8	3.3	3.9	4.4	4.9	5.5	6.0	6.5
14–16	3.2	3.8	4.3	4.8	5.4	5.9	6.4	7.0	7.5
17–19	4.2	4.7	5.3	5.8	6.3	6.9	7.4	8.0	8.5
20–22	5.1	5.7	6.2	6.8	7.3	7.9	8.4	8.9	9.5
23–25	6.1	6.6	7.2	7.7	8.3	8.8	9.4	9.9	10.5
26–28	7.0	7.6	8.1	8.7	9.2	9.8	10.3	10.9	11.4
29–31	8.0	8.5	9.1	9.6	10.2	10.7	11.3	11.8	12.4
32–34	8.9	9.4	10.0	10.5	11.1	11.6	12.2	12.8	13.3
35–37	9.8	10.4	10.9	11.5	12.0	12.6	13.1	13.7	14.3
38–40	10.7	11.3	11.8	12.4	12.9	13.5	14.1	14.6	15.2
41–43	11.6	12.2	12.7	13.3	13.8	14.4	15.0	15.5	16.1
44–46	12.5	13.1	13.6	14.2	14.7	15.3	15.9	16.4	17.0
47–49	13.4	13.9	14.5	15.1	15.6	16.2	16.8	17.3	17.9
50–52	14.3	14.8	15.4	15.9	16.5	17.1	17.6	18.2	18.8
53–55	15.1	15.7	16.2	16.8	17.4	17.9	18.5	19.1	19.7
56–58	16.0	16.5	17.1	17.7	18.2	18.8	19.4	20.0	20.5
59–61	16.9	17.4	17.9	18.5	19.1	19.7	20.2	20.8	21.4
62–64	17.6	18.2	18.8	19.4	19.9	20.5	21.1	21.7	22.2
65–67	18.5	19.0	19.6	20.2	20.8	21.3	21.9	22.5	23.1
68–70	19.3	19.9	20.4	21.0	21.6	22.2	22.7	23.3	23.9
71–73	20.1	20.7	21.2	21.8	22.4	23.0	23.6	24.1	24.7
74–76	20.9	21.5	22.0	22.6	23.2	23.8	24.4	25.0	25.5
77–79	21.7	22.2	22.8	23.4	24.0	24.6	25.2	25.8	26.3
80–82	22.4	23.0	23.6	24.2	24.8	25.4	25.9	26.5	27.1
83–85	23.2	23.8	24.4	25.0	25.5	26.1	26.7	27.3	27.9
86–88	24.0	24.5	25.1	25.7	26.3	26.9	27.5	28.1	28.7
89–91	24.7	25.3	25.9	25.5	27.1	27.6	28.2	28.8	29.4
92–94	25.4	26.0	26.6	27.2	27.8	28.4	29.0	29.6	30.2
95–97	26.1	26.7	27.3	27.9	28.5	29.1	29.7	30.3	30.9
98–100	26.9	27.4	28.0	28.6	29.2	29.8	30.4	31.0	31.6
101–103	27.5	28.1	28.7	29.3	29.9	30.5	31.1	31.7	32.3
104–106	28.2	28.8	29.4	30.0	30.6	31.2	31.8	32.4	33.0
107–109	28.9	29.5	30.1	30.7	31.3	31.9	32.5	33.1	33.7
110–112	29.6	30.2	30.8	31.4	32.0	32.6	33.2	33.8	34.4
113–115	30.2	30.8	31.4	32.0	32.6	33.2	33.8	34.5	35.1

*Percent fat calculated by the Siri Formula: (% fat = [4.95/BD-4.5] × 100), where BD = body density.

**Taken from Pollock, M. L., Schmidt, D. H., and Jackson, A. S. "Measurement of Cardiorespiration Fitness and Body Composition in the Clinical Setting." *Comprehensive Therapy,* Vol. 6, September 1980.

TABLE 7.3* Percent fat estimates for women using the sum of the triceps, iliac crest, and thigh skinfolds.**

Female Sum of Skin Folds (mm)	<23	Age 23 to 27	28 to 32	33 to 37	38 to 42	43 to 47	48 to 52	53 to 57	Over 58
23–25	9.7	9.9	10.2	10.4	10.7	10.9	11.2	11.4	11.7
26–28	11.0	11.2	11.5	11.7	12.0	12.3	12.5	12.7	13.0
29–31	12.3	12.5	12.8	13.0	13.3	13.5	13.8	14.0	14.3
32–34	13.6	13.8	14.0	14.3	14.5	14.8	15.0	15.3	15.5
35–37	14.8	15.0	15.3	15.5	15.8	16.0	16.3	16.5	16.8
38–40	16.0	16.3	16.5	16.7	17.0	17.2	17.5	17.7	18.0
41–43	17.2	17.4	17.7	17.9	18.2	18.4	18.7	18.9	19.2
44–46	18.3	18.6	18.8	19.1	19.3	19.6	19.8	20.1	20.3
47–49	19.5	19.7	20.0	20.2	20.5	20.7	21.0	21.2	21.5
50–52	20.6	20.8	21.1	21.3	21.6	21.8	22.1	22.3	22.6
53–55	21.7	21.9	22.1	22.4	22.6	22.9	23.1	23.4	23.6
56–58	22.7	23.0	23.2	23.4	23.7	23.9	24.2	24.4	24.7
59–61	23.7	24.0	24.2	24.5	24.7	25.0	25.2	25.5	25.7
62–64	24.7	25.0	25.2	25.5	35.7	26.0	26.7	26.4	26.7
65–67	25.7	25.9	26.2	26.4	26.7	26.9	27.2	27.4	27.7
68–70	26.6	26.9	27.1	27.4	27.6	27.9	28.1	28.4	28.6
71–73	27.5	27.8	28.0	28.3	28.5	28.8	28.0	29.3	29.5
74–76	28.4	28.7	28.0	28.3	28.5	29.7	29.9	30.2	30.4
77–79	29.3	29.5	29.8	30.0	30.3	30.5	30.8	31.0	31.3
80–82	30.1	30.4	30.6	30.9	31.1	31.4	31.6	31.9	32.1
83–85	30.9	31.2	31.4	31.7	31.9	32.2	32.4	32.7	32.9
86–88	31.7	32.0	32.2	32.5	32.7	32.9	33.2	33.4	33.7
89–91	32.5	32.7	33.0	33.2	33.5	33.7	33.9	34.2	34.4
92–94	33.2	33.4	33.7	33.9	34.2	34.4	34.7	34.9	35.2
95–97	33.9	34.1	34.4	34.6	34.9	35.1	35.4	35.6	35.9
98–100	34.6	34.8	35.1	35.3	35.5	35.8	36.0	36.3	36.5
101–103	35.3	35.4	35.7	35.9	36.2	36.4	36.7	36.9	37.2
104–106	35.8	36.1	36.3	36.6	36.8	37.1	37.3	37.5	37.8
107–109	36.4	36.7	36.9	37.1	37.4	37.6	37.9	38.1	38.4
110–112	37.0	37.2	37.5	37.7	38.0	38.2	38.5	38.7	38.9
113–115	37.5	37.8	38.0	38.2	38.5	38.7	39.0	39.2	39.5

*Percent fat calculated by the Siri Formula: (% fat = [4.95/BD-4.5] × 100], where BD = body density.

**Taken from Pollock, M. L., Schmidt, D. H., and Jackson, A. S. "Measurement of Cardiorespiration Fitness and Body Composition in the Clinical Setting." *Comprehensive Therapy,* Vol. 6, September 1980.

Many factors influence the control of body weight. These factors include:

Genetic Predisposition	+	Activity	+	Eating Habits	=	Weight
metabolic rate		work		types of food		same
number & type of		leisure		quantities		lose
fat cells		exercise		location		gain
sex				attitudes		
				moods		

Genetic Predisposition.   The average American becomes more sedentary during the adult years. This leads to a decrease in lean muscle tissue and a decline in the metabolic rate. If your caloric intake is not reduced as the metabolic rate decreases, creeping obesity will occur. Creeping obesity, a form of obesity that occurs slowly over a period of several years, tends to be offset by an active lifestyle.

It is believed that the metabolic rate can be controlled in an attempt to maintain an ideal biological weight (the setpoint) by a body weight and fat regulating mechanism located in the hypothalamus of the brain. This ideal biological weight is different for each individual. Apparently, the mechanism responds to both calories and nutrients. When the caloric intake is restricted, your body attempts to maintain the present weight and fat by lowering the metabolic rate. Also, when sufficient amounts of certain nutrients are not consumed, your appetite increases. This setpoint is thought to be one of the primary reasons some people have such a hard time losing weight without gaining it back. According to the setpoint theory, the key to controlling weight is to control the setpoint. Lowering the setpoint can be accomplished through any of the following: (1) exercise; (2) a diet high in complex carbohydrates; (3) nicotine; and (4) amphetamines. Since nicotine and amphetamines have a destructive effect upon the body, the most effective way to lower the setpoint is through exercise combined with a diet high in complex carbohydrates.

There are two types of fat cells in the body—yellow and brown. The yellow fat cells are predominant and comprise approximately 99% of the total fat cells in the body. The number of yellow fat cells can be altered by diet and exercise during infancy and adolescence. Excessive caloric intake tends to promote yellow fat cell production in the formative years which, in turn, determines the ability of the body to store fat throughout life. To curb this potential for unnecessary yellow fat cell production, preventative steps need to be taken at an early age through proper nutritional and exercise habits. In light of what is now known about yellow fat cell production, the saying *"a fat baby is a healthy baby"* seems inappropriate.

Brown fat cells contain a high amount of the iron-containing hemoglobin pigment found in red blood cells. Instead of storing fat, it is thought that brown fat cells have the capacity to produce as much as 25% to 50% of the body's heat by burning fat. The number of brown fat cells appears to be genetically determined and not affected by exercise or diet. The number of brown fat cells varies from individual to individual. This helps explain why some individuals simply do not gain weight.

Activity Levels.   In today's society, many of the physically demanding jobs of the past are now performed by machines. This automation has helped us to develop a much more sedentary lifestyle than at any time in history. Even sedentary leisure activities have become popular in this new era of microelectronics; many individuals have replaced vigorous activities such as cycling, hiking, and swimming with passive activities such as watching television and playing computer games. As Americans have become more sedentary, they have also become less fit and more overfat.

Another problem facing Americans is the physical education requirement in the public school systems. Recent studies have shown that youth are less fit today than they were a decade ago. In many schools, students experience vigorous activity only once a week, if at all. This is not sufficient to gain an adequate level of fitness. In fact, research now indicates the average adult between 30 and 40 years of age is more fit than his or her teen-age counterpart. Hopefully, as Americans become better educated about the benefits of exercise with regard to fitness and weight control, this trend will be reversed.

Eating Habits. The eating habits you develop are an important part of your weight control program. These habits relate not only to the types of food you eat, but also to when, how, and how much you eat. Research has indicated that overfat individuals tend to be more susceptible to external cues. External cues are environmental factors—other than true hunger—that may trigger you to eat. You may associate eating with watching television, reading, or listening to music. Significant emotional changes, such as anxiety or depression, may also contribute to overeating as a method to abate psychological distress. Other behavioral factors that may lead to significant weight gain are eating late at night before bedtime, high calorie snacking, and eating rapidly. Besides increasing your caloric intake, diets high in fats, refined carbohydrates, and artificial sweeteners are thought to raise the setpoint. Eliminating some of these adverse eating habits is best done through behavior modification, which allows you to recognize poor eating habits and change them through a relearning process. The University of North Carolina at Chapel Hill has identified some tips for eating and shopping. These include:

1. Decide to make eating a "pure" experience by engaging in no other activities while eating besides socializing with family and friends (i.e., no reading, TV, etc.).
2. Do all of your eating in the kitchen or dining room and then only while sitting down at your personal place at the table or counter.
3. Eliminate snacks.
4. Plan and record what you eat before you eat.
5. Pause for at least two to five minutes before beginning to eat.
6. Slow your rate of eating by placing utensils on your plate after every mouthful and not picking them up again until the food has been swallowed.
7. Measure every portion you take.
8. Make normal portions appear to be larger by using a smaller plate.
9. Make second helpings difficult to get.
10. Identify the people who are most likely to be of help to you. Inform them about your specific plans. Enlist their positive support.
11. Drink a glass of water ten minutes before each meal.
12. Eat whole fruit rather than drinking juice. It takes longer and is more satisfying.

13. Eat three small meals a day rather than two large meals.

14. Practice stocking only healthy low-caloric snacks in your refrigerator.

15. Prepare a list of needed items before you enter the store and buy nothing that is not on your list.

16. Shop after you have eaten a full meal.

17. Avoid browsing! Walk only through the aisles that stock the foods you need.

18. Choose to buy non-problem foods.

19. If you feel you must buy problem foods, buy them in a form that requires the greatest possible level of preparation in the smallest possible portions.

20. Store all foods in covered containers that are kept only in the kitchen.

Eating Disorders. The current emphasis on physical appearance in our society has increased the frequency of eating disorders. Anorexia nervosa is now and has long been considered a serious problem. In the last several years bulimia has begun to occur with increasing frequency. Both are complex emotional disorders that could affect your psychological and physical well being.

Anorexia nervosa is a condition characterized by deliberate self starvation with profound pyschiatric and physical side effects. Common warning signs include: (1) an intense fear of becoming obese which does not diminish with increased weight loss and is sometimes accompanied by a distorted body image; (2) prolonged exercise in spite of fatigue, weakness, and hyperactivity; (3) at least a 25% loss of original body weight without some other illness accounting for the weight loss; (4) insisting on keeping one's body weight below the minimal level for age and height norms regardless of existing percent body fat; (5) unusual eating rituals or patterns.

Bulimia is characterized by food obsession with compulsive binge eating and purging. Binge eating is a rapid consumption of food in a short period of time. In a two hour period as much as 1000 to 55000 calories may be consumed, with the average consumption approximately 4800 calories. Often the binge consists of high caloric, easily ingested sweet food. In addition, the individual is normally secretive about the disorder. The termination of the binge is usually caused by abdominal pain, sleep, social interruption, or self-induced vomiting. Along with self-induced vomiting, the bulimic individual sometimes resorts to severely restrictive diets, laxatives, and diuretics as a means of losing weight. Because of the frequent alternation of bingeing, purging, and fasting, the bulimic individual experiences frequent weight fluctuations of as much as ten pounds. The individual is aware that the eating pattern is abnormal but is unable to stop eating. Often low self-esteem, stress and depression accompany the eating binges. It is interesting to note that the bulimic individual's body weight is often normal or slightly higher than normal.

Some individuals exhibit behavior patterns that are a combination of anorexia nervosa and bulimia. These disorders appear to be more common in women than in men. The causes of these eating disorders are not readily apparent; however, certain psychological factors do play a role. These include: (1) stressful life situations with which the individual is unable to cope; (2) concessions to excessive cultural pressure that often boasts that "thin is in"; (3) family gatherings centered around food; (4) the absence of meaningful peer relationships.

A positive approach for the treatment of anorexia nervosa and bulimia is a combination of medical treatment and psychotherapy for the patient and counseling for family members. Early detection and treatment is imperative for controlling these disorders. Unfortunately, some anorexic and bulimic individuals die as a result of their disorders. Some struggle with the condition for a lifetime while others recover with no further difficulty. Professional help for both anorexia nervosa and bulimia is available at most student health and counseling centers.

Preventing Obesity

Controlling your body fat and weight is a lifelong process of monitoring your diet, exercise, and eating habits. There are no easy ways to control your weight. Drugs, fancy gadgets, surgery, and drastic diets seem to promise the world to those who are desperate, but their results and safety are questionable. It is believed that the most intelligent and effective method of maintaining your ideal weight and combating obesity is to eat a sensible diet and exercise on a regular basis.

Role of Exercise.   Exercise plays an important part in the battle against obesity. Dieters too often concentrate solely on dieting and neglect the role that increased physical activity can play in a weight reduction program. The weight loss one experiences during a weight control program consists of both fat weight and lean muscle mass. With dieting alone, approximately 30% of the total weight loss will be lean muscle mass. However, when exercise is combined with dieting, only 5% to 10% of the weight loss is lean muscle mass.

Much evidence supports the theory that physical inactivity is the factor most responsible for the increasing number of overfat people in modern Western societies. Several studies, comparing food intake and physical activity patterns of overfat individuals, attributed the fat weight difference to a sedentary lifestyle instead of food consumption—the food intake was not significantly different for those who were overfat and those who were not. The forms of exercise found to be most helpful in a weight reducing program were activities that demanded large caloric expenditures such as slow, long distance running. Table 7.4 lists numerous activities and the caloric expenditure for each. If a weight training program is used, the exercises should be performed with light resistance and high repetitions.

In addition to maintaining a higher level of lean muscle mass, exercise plays other important roles in your weight control program. Training at least four times per week for a duration of thirty minutes per training session appears to lower the setpoint. This allows you to lose and then maintain a lower body weight and body fat percentage. Also, during vigorous exercise, your metabolic rate may increase as much as thirteen times the resting rate. Your body weight and duration of the exercise is more important for caloric expenditure than the intensity level. Table 7.5 shows that a person who weighs 150 pounds and runs three miles in sixteen minutes will burn only sixteen more calories than by running the same distance in twenty four minutes (310 versus 294 calories). Another point that needs to be emphasized is the caloric expenditure during recovery from exer-

TABLE 7.4 Activity and caloric expenditure.

Activity (½ hour)	120 lb. Female	160 lb. Male
Badminton	180–220	220–260
Baseball	160–200	200–240
Basketball	300–400	400–600
Bicycling moderately	100–120	120–140
Bicyling energetically	200–230	280–320
Bowling	80–120	100–140
Canoeing	100–150	130–180
Carpentry, workbench	120–140	140–180
Climbing stairs	130–160	160–190
Cooking, active	60–90	80–110
Dancing, moderately	100–130	130–170
Dancing, energetically, disco	200–400	250–500
Dishwashing, by hand	60–90	80–110
Dressing, undressing	30–50	35–60
Driving, auto	50–60	60–75
Exercising moderately	140–170	180–220
Exercising energetically	200–250	250–350
Football	250–300	300–400
Gardening, active	120–140	140–180
Golf, no cart	100–140	130–170
Golf, with cart	70–90	80–110
Handball	200–350	300–400
Hockey, field, ice	250–350	300–400
Horseback riding	140–160	160–200
Housework, active	80–130	110–160
Jogging, light	200–250	250–300
Lying, sitting, at rest	15–20	20–25
Office work, active	70–130	90–150
Reading	15–20	20–25
Rowing vigorously	300–400	400–500
Running	300–400	400–500
Sawing wood	250–300	300–400
Sewing	25–30	30–35
Skating energetically	200–300	250–300
Soccer	250–350	350–400
Squash	180–240	250–400
Standing, relaxed	20–25	25–30
Swimming steadily	200–300	300–400
Table tennis	150–180	200–250
Tennis, amateur	180–220	250–280
Volleyball	180–220	220–280
Walking moderately	80–100	90–120
Walking energetically	140–160	160–180
Writing	25–80	30–100

Adapted from *The Complete Scarsdale Medical Diet,* by Herman Tarnower and Samm Baker.

cise. As mentioned earlier, if a 150 pound person ran three miles in twenty four minutes, 294 calories would be expended. However, the metabolic rate would be increased an additional thirty to fifty calories per hour for the next six to eight hours. This would result in an additional 180 to 400 calories being expended and therefore the total caloric expenditure would be approximately 474 to 694 calories.

TABLE 7.5 Caloric values for running 3 miles at various speeds.

Weight in lbs.		Running time: minutes								
		16	18	20	22	24	26	28	30	32
120	C>	250	248	242	240	238	234	232	228	224
130	A>	270	266	264	260	256	252	250	246	242
140	L>	290	286	282	278	276	272	268	264	260
150	O>	310	306	302	298	294	290	286	282	278
160	R>	330	326	322	318	312	308	304	300	296
170	I>	350	346	340	336	332	328	322	318	314
180	E>	370	364	360	356	350	346	342	336	332
190	S>	390	384	380	374	370	363	360	354	350

Guidelines for Proper Weight Reduction

It is estimated that sixty to seventy million American adults and at least ten million American teenagers are obese. Since millions of Americans have adopted unsupervised weight loss programs, it is the opinion of the American College of Sports Medicine that guidelines are needed. Therefore, the American College of Sports Medicine has issued the following statements as guidelines to your weight reduction program.

1. Prolonged fasting and diet programs that severely restrict caloric intake are scientifically undesirable and can be medically dangerous due to the loss of large amounts of water, electrolytes, minerals, glycogen stores, and other fat-free tissue (including proteins within fat-free tissues).

2. Mild caloric restriction (500 to 1000 calories less than the usual daily intake) results in a smaller loss of water, electrolytes, minerals, and other fat-free tissue, and is less likely to cause malnutrition.

3. Dynamic exercise of large muscles (such as running, swimming, cycling, handball, and racquetball) helps to maintain fat-free tissue, including muscle mass and bone density, and results in loss of body weight. Weight loss resulting from an increase in energy expenditure is primarily in the form of fat weight.

4. A nutritionally sound diet resulting in mild caloric restriction combined with an endurance exercise program is recommended for weight reduction. The rate of sustained weight loss should not exceed two pounds per week.

5. To maintain proper weight control and optimal body fat levels, a lifetime commitment to proper eating habits and regular physical activity is required.

Commonly Asked Questions About Weight Control

The following are questions commonly asked by individuals attempting to control body weight and body fat.

1. *Is it possible to spot reduce?* Spot reducing is possible only through surgery. When weight loss occurs in the body, fat is lost from all areas where fat is stored. However, the areas of the body with the greater amount of fat will have the greater percentage of fat loss.

2. *Is crash dieting dangerous?* Yes! Crash dieting implies a radical reduction in food consumption bordering on semi-starvation. A major problem with this type of weight loss is that essential proteins, vitamins, and minerals are eliminated from the diet. Also, a large part of the weight loss from crash diets consists of protein and water from lean muscle tissue, which is replaced rapidly when eating is resumed. Most physicians agree that excess fat should be removed from the body the same way it was deposited—slowly and gradually. A reduction of two pounds per week is considered both safe and practical.

3. *Does muscle turn to fat when one stops exercising?* No, muscle does not turn to fat when one stops exercising or at any other time. However, belief in this myth is easy to understand when one observes a once lean, muscular individual who has become fat and flabby since his or her training days. What appears to be muscle changing to fat is simply the cumulative effects of long term deconditioning and a positive caloric imbalance. The muscle cells atrophy due to inactivity as the fat cells increase in size due to the caloric intake being greater than the caloric expenditure.

4. *Does exercise increase one's appetite?* Some overfat people are apprehensive about using exercise to help reduce body fat because they are afraid exercise will increase their appetite and thus cause them to gain more bodyfat. However, this is not the case. Human beings were intended to be active beings. Initially, vigorous activity suppresses the appetite. After a period of time, appetite may increase but it is not proportional to the increased caloric expenditure resulting from the increased activity.

5. *Is it true that the amount of energy required to burn one pound of fat is equal to walking 35 miles or chopping wood for seven hours?* Yes, this is true. However, it is important to put these assertions into proper perspective. Walking a mile a day for 35 days or chopping wood for fifteen minutes per day for a month will also take off one pound of body fat. Also, remember the caloric expenditure during recovery is not being considered in the above example.

In summary, many factors should be considered when attempting to control your body weight and percent body fat. Good eating habits, proper diet, and a vigorous exercise program all go hand in hand in this effort.

Supplementary Readings

1. Blumenthal, James, S. Rose, and J. Chang. "Anorexia Nervosa and Exercise." *Sports Medicine,* No. 2, 1985.

2. D'Augelli, A. R., and W. H. Smiciklas. "The Case for Primary Prevention of Overweight through the Family." *Journal of Nutrition Education,* April–June 1978.

3. Epstein, L. H., and R. R. Wing. "Aerobic Exercise and Weight." *Addictive Behavior,* Vol. 5, 1980.

4. Goodhart, R. S., and M. E. Shils, eds. *Modern Nutrition in Health & Disease.* Philadelphia, PA: Lea and Febiger, 1988.

5. Guyton, A. C. *Textbook of Medical Physiology.* New York: Saunders College Publishing, 1986.

6. Hager, A. "Nutritional Problems in Adolescence—Obesity." *Nutrition Reviews,* February 1981.

7. Hanna, C. H., et al. "Differences in the Degree of Overweight: A Note of Its Importance." *Addictive Behaviors,* 1981.

8. Hargetetal, B. S. "The Caloric Cost of Running." *Journal of American Medical Association,* Vol. 8, 1974.

9. Hertzler, A. A. "Obesity—Impact on Family." *Journal of the American Dietetic Association,* November 1981.

10. Keys, A. "Overweight, Obesity, Coronary Heart Disease and Mortality." *Nutrition Reviews,* September 1980.

11. Marley, W. P. *Health and Physical Fitness.* Dubuque, IA: Wm. C. Brown, 1988.

12. Metropolitan Life Insurance Company. "New Weight Standards for Men and Women." *Statistical Bulletin,* 1983.

13. Neuman, P. A., and P. A. Halvorson. *Anorexia Nervosa and Bulimia.* New York: Van Nostrand Reinhold Company, 1983.

14. Rodin, J., and J. Slochower. "Externality in the Nonobese: Effects of Environmental Responsiveness on Weight." *Journal of Personality and Social Psychology,* Vol. 33, 1976.

15. University of North Carolina Health Services. *Aids for Eating More Sensibly,* February 1981.

8
Stress Management

During the course of any day you are required to make a number of decisions while preparing for exams, meeting deadlines on projects, getting a date for the football game, or living with an unbearable roommate. These are situations normally experienced by college students; however, though they are normal they may also be stressful. Today people are subjected to an ever increasing amount of stress.

What Is Stress?

The term *stress* has many definitions. Some researchers define stress as anything that threatens the existence of an organism. Others describe stress as an upset of the homeostatic balance of the body caused by psychic, physical, or social conditions. A moderate level of stress is desirable—it prepares the body to react to the stress-causing event and will improve performance. However, too much stress will result in a decrease in performance and health. Stress can have a positive effect or negative effect, depending upon your ability to cope.

Physical Responses to Stress

How does the body respond to stressful situations? The bodily responses to stress vary among individuals. Different emotional states activate the release of epinephrine and norepinephrine from the adrenal medulla. These hormones can increase the body's capacity to perform vigorous muscular activity by (1) increasing arterial pressure; (2) increasing blood flow to the active muscles and decreasing the blood flow to organs not needed for rapid activity; (3) increasing the rates of cellular metabolism throughout the body; (4) increasing the blood glucose concentration; (5) increasing glycolysis in the muscle; (6) increasing muscular strength; (7) increasing mental activity; and (8) increasing the rate of blood coagulation. These are positive adaptive responses triggered by different stimuli. However, if these responses are not immediately followed by vigorous exercise, a number of negative things can happen to the body. These include: (1) constant low-level strain on the cardiovascular system that can lead to heart disease; (2) increased level of cholesterol combined with a decreased ability to clear the blood of this cholesterol; and (3) an increased tendency for the clotting elements of the blood to fall out and settle onto the walls of the veins and arteries. Vigorous muscular activity will enhance the conversion of fatty acids into energy before they collect along the arterials walls. However, lack of vigorous muscular activity increases the chances of atherosclerosis developing.

Physical cues often signal the onset of stress in individuals; these cues may vary from one person to another. Tightening of neck muscles, minor headaches, or an upset stomach may be experienced. Other physical responses include loss of appetite, inability to sleep, and a disruption of bodily functions. In addition, if you are continually aroused by stress, you are more likely to develop high blood pressure, ulcers, diabetes, and colitis.

Behavioral Patterns

The behavioral patterns you develop may have a positive or negative influence on the way that you handle stress. Generally, behavioral patterns are broken into three classes, which we'll call Types A, B, and C.

Type A individuals are typically over-achievers, excessively competitive, constantly impatient, hard driving, high-strung, and harbor free floating hostility. On the other hand, Type B individuals are usually relaxed, easy going, and casual. The traits of the Type B individual are almost exactly opposite those of the Type A individual. Type C individuals possess the same traits as Type A except they do not harbor feelings of hostility.

Until recently, there was no distinction between Type A and Type C behavior. Epidemiologists realized that people who were Type A had a much higher incidence of coronary heart disease than did Type B. However, these were the Type A individuals with feelings of anger and hostility. Those without feelings of anger and hostility had incidence rates of coronary heart disease comparable to their Type B counterparts. These individuals have been reclassified as Type C. These individuals normally are hard driving, highly competitive, over achievers, and often participate in a regular fitness program to keep themselves physically prepared for the demands placed upon them.

Managing Stress

Understanding your behavior patterns and realizing that stress can exact a severe toll on your health are important factors in behavior modification. It is thought that behavioral patterns, including those associated with Type A, are learned and developed.

To bring about a change in your ability to handle stress your perspective of life may need to be altered. How you perceive life's situations determines whether an event is stressful to you or not. Often two individuals will view the same event in different ways; one individual may experience a high level of stress while the other may experience very little stress. The example of two students preparing for an English exam might be used to demonstrate this point. One approaches the exam as a necessary step in his preparation to become an engineer. The second student is upset about the exam—he perceives it as a waste of his time because his goal is to become an engineer, not an English major. Both face the same task, but view it differently.

You cannot assume that others are responsible for your problems. Failure to take responsibility for your own problems will not solve them. There is merit in the old saying, "Look in a mirror and you can usually find both the cause and solution to your problems." To a great degree, we are what we want to be.

In your dealings with other people, try to be understanding and attempt to see the other person's point of view. Realize that most people have good reasons for their positions.

Develop the ability to look at the big picture. Often incidents may seem extremely important to you at the time they occur. However, attempt to analyze the incident in a larger time frame and usually it will appear less important and traumatic. An example of this may be an individual who fails at a given task. No one enjoys performing poorly. However, it will be less important as time passes. It is important to realize that you, like everyone else, are going to experience a few disappointments during life. You need to develop an appreciation for the simple things so that you will be able to handle the disappointments that you may experience. Take time each day to reflect upon life's gifts and beauty. Life is generally what we make of it.

Mental and muscle relaxation methods are used by some to eliminate stress. Mental relaxation may often be attained by finding a quiet place where you can sit or lie comfortably and close your eyes. Once in this position, listening to soothing music may help. Combining the mental relaxation techniques with muscular relaxation is often beneficial. The muscular relaxation method consists of attempting to tense a muscle group and then relaxing it. Start with your toes and work toward your head. Attempt to focus your attention on the soothing feeling of relaxation that follows the muscle tension. Each muscle group of the body should be relaxed this way. Breathing techniques are also used for relaxation. Slow deep breathing and sighing often bring relief from stress. Other methods for relaxation include meditation and self suggestion techniques.

Physical exercise may play a major role in helping to combat stress. The mind and the body are intimately linked with your health. Exercise is of great importance to the human body in managing stress. Vigorous exercise helps to relieve muscular tension and helps return the levels of epinephrine and norepinephrine back to normal. Many students use the early evening hours as their time for exercise in order to relieve the stress that mounts during the day. By dissipating the stress that you accumulated during the day, you are better able to handle your studies at night.

Anger or tension can often be converted to the satisfying feelings of sedation and fatigue that one experiences after sustained physical exertion. The feeling of anxiety that may be present before an upcoming event may be lessened by vigorous exercises. The physical benefits derived from exercise are just as important as the mental ones. Good muscle tone and an improved cardiovascular system will reduce the physiological problems that can develop as a result of stressful situations.

Measuring Stress and Tension

This is a four-part test developed by the Public Health Service of the former U.S. Department of Health, Education, and Welfare (now the Department of Health and Human Services). The first three parts are designed to give you an indication of how vulnerable you might be to certain types of stress and to make you aware of how they might affect you. The last part of the test will provide you with information on how to cope with situations that might be of a stressful nature. Additional information regarding this test can be found in DHEW Publication No. (PHS) 79-50097, Washington, D.C., 1980.

TEST ONE

Choose the most appropriate answer for each of the 10 questions as it actually pertains to you.

1. When I can't do something "my way," I simply adjust and do it the easiest way.
(a) Almost always true,   (b) Usually true,   (c) Usually false,   (d) Almost always false.

2. I get upset when someone in front of me drives slowly.
(a) Almost always true,   (b) Usually true,   (c) Usually false,   (d) Almost always false.

3. It bothers me when my plans are dependent upon others.
(a) Almost always true,   (b) Usually true,   (c) Usually false,   (d) Almost always false.

4. Whenever possible, I tend to avoid large crowds.
(a) Almost always true,   (b) Usually true,   (c) Usually false,   (d) Almost always false.

5. I am uncomfortable when I have to stand in long lines.
(a) Almost always true,   (b) Usually true,   (c) Usually false,   (d) Almost always false.

6. Arguments upset me.
(a) Almost always true,   (b) Usually true,   (c) Usually false,   (d) Almost always false.

7. When my plans don't flow smoothly, I become anxious.
(a) Almost always true,   (b) Usually true,   (c) Usually false,   (d) Almost always false.

8. I require a lot of space in which to live and work.
(a) Almost always true,   (b) Usually true,   (c) Usually false,   (d) Almost always false.

9. When I am busy at some task, I hate to be disturbed.
(a) Almost always true, (b) Usually true, (c) Usually false, (d) Almost always false.

10. I believe that it is worth waiting for all good things.
(a) Almost always true, (b) Usually true, (c) Usually false, (d) Almost always false.

To score: 1 and 10, a = 1 pt., b = 2 pts., c = 3 pts., d = 4 pts.; 2 through 9, a = 4 pts., b = 3 pts., c = 2 pts., d = 1 pt.

Test One measures your vulnerability to stress from being frustrated or inhibited. Scores in excess of 25 seem to suggest some vulnerability to this source of stress.

TEST TWO

Circle the letter of the response that best answers the following 10 questions. How often do you . . .

1. Find yourself with insufficient time to complete your work?
(a) Almost always, (b) Very often, (c) Seldom, (d) Never

2. Find yourself becoming confused and unable to think clearly because too many things are happening at once?
(a) Almost always, (b) Very often, (c) Seldom, (d) Never

3. Wish you had help to get everything done?
(a) Almost always, (b) Very often, (c) Seldom, (d) Never

4. Feel your boss/professor expects too much from you?
(a) Almost always, (b) Very often, (c) Seldom, (d) Never

5. Feel your family and friends expect too much from you?
(a) Almost always, (b) Very often, (c) Seldom, (d) Never

6. Find your work infringing on your leisure hours?
(a) Almost always, (b) Very often, (c) Seldom, (d) Never

7. Find yourself doing extra work to set an example to those around you?
(a) Almost always, (b) Very often, (c) Seldom, (d) Never

8. Find yourself doing extra work to impress your superiors?
(a) Almost always, (b) Very often, (c) Seldom, (d) Never

9. Have to skip a meal so that you can get work completed?
(a) Almost always, (b) Very often, (c) Seldom, (d) Never

10. Feel that you have too much responsibility?
(a) Almost always, (b) Very often, (c) Seldom, (d) Never

To score: a = 4 pts., b = 3 pts., c = 2 pts., d = 1 pt. Total your score for this exercise.

TEST THREE

Answer each question as it is generally true for you.

1. I hate to wait in lines.
   (a) Almost always true,   (b) Usually true,   (c) Seldom true,   (d) Never true

2. I often find myself racing against the clock to save time.
   (a) Almost always true,   (b) Usually true,   (c) Seldom true,   (d) Never true

3. I become upset if I think something is taking too long.
   (a) Almost always true,   (b) Usually true,   (c) Seldom true,   (d) Never true

4. When under pressure I tend to lose my temper.
   (a) Almost always true,   (b) Usually true,   (c) Seldom true,   (d) Never true

5. My friends tell me that I tend to get irritated easily.
   (a) Almost always true,   (b) Usually true,   (c) Seldom true,   (d) Never true

6. I seldom like to do anything unless I can make it competitive.
   (a) Almost always true,   (b) Usually true,   (c) Seldom true,   (d) Never true

7. When something must be done, I'm the first to begin even though the details may still need to be worked out.
   (a) Almost always true,   (b) Usually true,   (c) Seldom true,   (d) Never true

8. When I make a mistake it is usually because I've rushed into something without giving it enough thought and planning.
   (a) Almost always true,   (b) Usually true,   (c) Seldom true,   (d) Never true

9. Whenever possible, I try to do two things at once, such as eating while working, or planning while driving or bathing.
   (a) Almost always true,   (b) Usually true,   (c) Seldom true,   (d) Never true

10. When I go on a vacation, I usually take along some work to do just in case I get a chance.
    (a) Almost always true,   (b) Usually true,   (c) Seldom true,   (d) Never true

To score: a = 4 pts., b = 3 pts., c = 2 pts., d = 1 pt.

This test measures the presence of compulsive, time-urgent, and excessively aggressive behavioral traits. Scores in excess of 25 suggest the presence of one or more of these traits.

TEST FOUR

This test was created largely on the basis of results compiled by clinicians and researchers who sought to identify how individuals effectively cope with stress. This test is an educational tool, not a clinical instrument. Its purpose, therefore, is to inform you of ways in which you can effectively and healthfully cope with the stress in your life. At the same time, through a point system, it will give you some indication of the relative desirability of the coping strategies you are currently using. Simply follow the instructions given for each of the 14 items listed. Total your points when you have completed all of the items.

1. Give yourself 10 points if you feel that you have a supportive family.
2. Give yourself 10 points if you actively pursue a hobby.
3. Give yourself 10 points if you belong to some social or activity group that meets at least once a month (other than your family).
4. Give yourself 15 points if you are within five pounds of your ideal body weight, considering your height and bone structure.
5. Give yourself 15 points if you practice some form of deep relaxation at least three times a week. Deep relaxation exercises include meditation, imagery, yoga, and so on.
6. Give yourself 5 points for each time you exercise thirty minutes or longer during one average week.
7. Give yourself 5 points for each nutritionally balanced and wholesome meal you consume during one average day.
8. Give yourself 5 points if you do something just for yourself that you really enjoy during an average week.
9. Give yourself 10 points if you have some place in your home that you can go in order to relax and/or be alone.
10. Give yourself 10 points if you practice time management techniques in your daily life.
11. Subtract 10 points for each pack of cigarettes you smoke during one average day.
12. Subtract 5 points for each evening during an average week that you take any form of medication or chemical substance (including alcohol) to help you sleep.
13. Subtract 10 points for each day during an average week that you consume any form of medication or chemical substance (including alcohol) to reduce your anxiety or just to calm you down.
14. Subtract 5 points for each evening during an average week that you bring work home—work that was meant to be done at your place of employment.

Now calculate your total score. A "perfect" score would be 115 points or more. If you scored in the 50 to 60 range you probably have an adequate collection of coping strategies for most common sources of stress. You should keep in mind, however, that the higher your score, the greater your ability to cope with stress.

Supplementary Readings

1. Blumenthal, James. "Relaxation Therapy, Biofeedback, and Behavioral Medicine." *Psychotherapy,* Vol. 22, No. 3, 1985.

2. Blumenthal, James, S. Rose, and J. Chang. "Anorexia Nervosa and Exercise." *Sports Medicine,* No. 2, 1985.

3. Charlesworth, Edward, and R. Nathan. "How to Build a Healthy Response to Stress." *Advertizing Age,* Vol. 56, 1985.

4. *Duke Health Line,* Vol. 1, No. 1, 1985.

5. Gil, Karen, and J. Blumenthal. "Behavior Modification in the Primary and Secondary Prevention of Coronary Heart Disease." *Cardiology in Practice,* Vol. 1, No. 6, 1985.

6. Guyton, Arthur. *Textbook of Medical Physiology.* Philadelphia, PA: W. B. Saunders, 1986.

7. Kleiner, Brian, and S. Geil. "Managing Stress Effectively." *Journal of Systems Management,* 1985.

8. Kriegel, R. J., and M.H. Kriegel. *The C Zone: Peak Performance Under Stress.* Garden City, NY: Anchor Press/Doubleday, 1984.

9. Pascarella, Perry. "Job Stress: A State of Mind." *Industry Week,* Nov. 29, 1982.

Appendix A

Cardiorespiratory progress chart.

Name_____

Date	Type Exercise	Pre-exercise Heart Rate	Exercise Time	Target Heart Rate	Exercise Distance	Post-exercise Heart Rate	Goals

Cardiorespiratory progress chart.

Name_____

Date	Type Exercise	Pre-exercise Heart Rate	Exercise Time	Target Heart Rate	Exercise Distance	Post-exercise Heart Rate	Goals

Cardiorespiratory progress chart.

Name_____

Date	Type Exercise	Pre-exercise Heart Rate	Exercise Time	Target Heart Rate	Exercise Distance	Post-exercise Heart Rate	Goals

Appendix B

After

Weight
Right Bicep
Left Bicep
Chest Inf.
Chest Def.
Waist
Right Thigh
Left Thigh
% Fat

Before

Weight
Right Bicep
Left Bicep
Chest Inf.
Chest Def.
Waist
Right Thigh
Left Thigh
% Fat

Name _____

Class _____

Dates

Exercises

SET

	W	R	W	R	W	R	W	R	W	R	W	R	W	R	W	R	W	R	W	R	W	R	W	R
1																								
2																								
3																								

Name ______________________

Class ______________________

Before

Weight	
Right Bicep	
Left Bicep	
Chest Inf.	
Chest Def.	
Waist	
Right Thigh	
Left Thigh	
% Fat	

After

Weight	
Right Bicep	
Left Bicep	
Chest Inf.	
Chest Def.	
Waist	
Right Thigh	
Left Thigh	
% Fat	

Dates																									
Exercises	SET	W	R	W	R	W	R	W	R	W	R	W	R	W	R	W	R	W	R	W	R	W	R	W	R
	1																								
	2																								
	3																								
	1																								
	2																								
	3																								
	1																								
	2																								
	3																								
	1																								
	2																								
	3																								
	1																								
	2																								
	3																								
	1																								
	2																								
	3																								
	1																								
	2																								
	3																								
	1																								
	2																								
	3																								
	1																								
	2																								
	3																								
	1																								
	2																								
	3																								

Name

Class

Before

Weight
Right Bicep
Left Bicep
Chest Inf.
Chest Def.
Waist
Right Thigh
Left Thigh
% Fat

After

Weight
Right Bicep
Left Bicep
Chest Inf.
Chest Def.
Waist
Right Thigh
Left Thigh
% Fat

Dates

Exercises

SET

SET	W	R	W	R	W	R	W	R	W	R	W	R	W	R	W	R	W	R	W	R	W	R	W	R	W	R
1																										
2																										
3																										
1																										
2																										
3																										
1																										
2																										
3																										
1																										
2																										
3																										
1																										
2																										
3																										
1																										
2																										
3																										
1																										
2																										
3																										

Index